USP – the standard of drug quality.

You may have seen the initials "USP" on the label of a drug product. They assure that legal standards of strength, quality, purity, packaging, and labeling exist for the medicine inside the package. What lies behind those initials is the United States Pharmacopeial Convention, Inc. (USP), a nongovernmental, nonprofit, unbiased scientific organization dedicated to quality health care.

The USP is made up of an elected body of representatives from colleges and national and state organizations of medicine and pharmacy. Since 1820 it has established the drug standards in the U.S. The USP standards are recognized as official by the Federal Food, Drug, and Cosmetic Act and are enforced by the U.S. Food and Drug Administration (FDA).

USP publishes the drug standards in the *United States Pharmacopeia* and the *National Formulary*. Additionally, the USP maintains a vast database of drug use information for both health care professionals and consumers, which is published as *USP DI*.® The information included in the "About Your Medicines" books is derived from the *USP DI* database.

For more information about USP see page viii.

About Your High Blood Pressure MEDICINES

By authority of the
United States Pharmacopeial Convention, Inc.
in cooperation with
The National High Blood Pressure Education Program

NOTICE AND WARNING

Concerning U.S. Patent or Trademark Rights

The inclusion in *About Your High Blood Pressure Medicines* of a monograph on any drug in respect to which patent or trademark rights may exist shall not be deemed, and is not intended as, a grant of, or authority to exercise, any right or privilege protected by such patent or trademark. All such rights and privileges are vested in the patent or trademark owner, and no other person may exercise the same without express permission, authority, or license secured from such patent or trademark owner.

The listing of selected brand names is intended only for ease of reference. The inclusion of a brand name does not mean the USPC has any particular knowledge that the brand listed has properties different from other brands of the same drug, nor should it be interpreted as an endorsement by the USPC. Similarly, the fact that a particular brand has not been included does not indicate that the product has been judged to be unsatisfactory or unacceptable.

Concerning Use of *About Your High Blood Pressure Medicines*

NOTICE: The information about the drugs contained herein is general in nature and is intended to be used in consultation with your health care providers. It is not intended to replace specific instructions or directions or warnings given to you by your physician or other prescriber or accompanying a particular product. The information is selective and it is not claimed that it includes all known precautions, contraindications, effects, or interactions possibly related to the use of a drug. The information may differ from that contained in the product labeling which is required by law. The information is not sufficient to make an evaluation as to the risks and benefits of taking a particular drug in a particular case and is not medical advice for individual problems and should not alone be relied upon for these purposes. Since the inclusion or exclusion of particular information about a drug is judgmental in nature and since opinion as to drug usage may differ, you may wish to consult additional sources. Should you desire additional information or if you have any questions as to how this information may relate to you in particular, ask your doctor, nurse, pharmacist, or other health care provider.

Printed by George Banta Company, Inc., Menasha, WI   54952.
Distributed by USPC, 12601 Twinbrook Pkwy., Rockville, MD   20852.

Contents

Introduction

Organization of This Book

The purpose of this book is to provide information about medicines used in the treatment of high blood pressure. Individual discussions (monographs) of these medicines begin on page 1 and are arranged in alphabetical order by generic name only. By looking in the Index, however, you can find either the brand name or the generic name of your medicine and the page listing for the monograph.

Preceding the drug monographs, there is a general discussion of high blood pressure and its treatment and general information about use of medicines. Clip-out treatment aids such as medication calendars, order forms for consumer materials, and wallet diaries are placed after the drug monographs as appendixes.

About USP

The information in this volume is prepared by the United States Pharmacopeial Convention, Inc. (USPC), the organization that sets the official standards of strength, quality, purity, packaging, and labeling for medical products used in the United States.

The United States Pharmacopeial Convention is an independent, nonprofit corporation composed of delegates from the accredited colleges of medicine and pharmacy in the U.S.; state medical and pharmaceutical associations; many national associations concerned with medicines, such as the American Medical Association, the American Nurses Association, the American Dental Association, the National Association of Retail Druggists (NARD), and the American Pharmaceutical Association; and various departments of the federal government, including the

Food and Drug Administration. In addition, four members of the Convention have been appointed by the Board of Trustees specifically to represent the public. USPC was established over 160 years ago, and is the only national body that represents the professions of both pharmacy and medicine.

The first convention came into being on January 1, 1820, and within the year published the first national drug formulary of the United States. The *United States Pharmacopeia* of 1820 contained 217 drug names, divided into two groups according to the level of general acceptance and usage.

When Congress passed the first major drug safety law in 1906, the standards recognized by that statute were those set forth in the *United States Pharmacopeia* and in the *National Formulary*. Today, the *USP* and *NF* continue to be the official U.S. compendia for standards for drugs and for the inactive ingredients in drug dosage forms. The *United States Pharmacopeia* is the world's oldest regularly revised national pharmacopeia and is generally accepted as being the most influential.

The work of the USPC is carried out by the Committee of Revision. This committee of experts is elected by the Convention and currently consists of 95 outstanding physicians, pharmacists, dentists, nurses, chemists, microbiologists, and other individuals particularly qualified to judge the merits of drugs and the standards and information that should apply to them. Committee members serve without pay and are assisted by numerous advisory panels, other outside reviewers, and USPC staff.

The monographs contained in *About Your High Blood Pressure Medicines* are extracted from *USP Dispensing Information (USP DI)*.

Three years in the making, the first annual edition of *USP DI* was published in 1980. It is a continuously reviewed and revised base of drug information intended for use by prescribers, dispensers, and consumers of medications. The information is developed by the consensus of the USP Committee of Revision and its Advisory Panels and anyone, including ordinary citizens, may contribute through review and comment on drafts of the monographs published in *USP DI Review*.

For further information about *USP DI* or if you have any comments as to how the information published in this volume might better meet your information needs, please contact: USP Drug Information Division, 12601 Twinbrook Parkway, Rockville, MD 20852 (301) 881-0666.

The United States Pharmacopeial Convention 1985–1990

William J. Keller, Ph.D.
(1985–1988)
Monroe, LA

B.J. Kennedy, M.D.
Minneapolis, MN

Jay S. Keystone, M.D.
Toronto, Ontario, Canada

Boen T. Kho, Ph.D.
Plattsburgh, NY

Lewis J. Leeson, Ph.D.
Summit, NJ

Herbert Letterman, Ph.D.
(1988–)
Somerville, NJ

Robert D. Lindeman, M.D.
Washington, DC

Charles H. Lochmuller, Ph.D.
Durham, NC

Dean H. Lockwood, M.D.
Rochester, NY

Jennifer M. H. Loggie, M.D.
Cincinnati, OH

Edward G. Lovering, Ph.D.
Ottawa, Ontario, Canada

John R. Markus, B.S.
Rockville, MD

Robert A. Mathews, Ph.D.
(1985–1986)
Washington, DC

Warren A. McAllister, Ph.D.
Greenville, NC

Thomas Medwick, Ph.D.
Piscataway, NJ

Robert F. Morrissey, Ph.D.
Somerville, NJ

Terry E. Munson
Fairfax, VA

Harold R. Nace, Ph.D.
Barrington, RI

Wendel L. Nelson, Ph.D.
Seattle, WA

Sharon C. Northup, Ph.D.
(1986–)
Round Lake, IL

Stanley P. Owen, Ph.D.
Federal Way, WA

James W. Pate, M.D.
Memphis, TN

Garnet E. Peck, Ph.D.
West Lafayette, IN

Robert V. Petersen, Ph.D.
Salt Lake City, UT

James R. Rankin, B.S.
Taos, NM

Christopher T. Rhodes, Ph.D.
Kingston, RI

Jay Roberts, Ph.D.
Philadelphia, PA

Joseph R. Robinson, Ph.D.
Madison, WI

Theodore J. Roseman, Ph.D.
Morton Grove, IL

Leonard P. Rybak, M.D., Ph.D.
Springfield, IL

Andrew J. Schmitz, Jr., M.S.
New York, NY

Stephen G. Schulman, Ph.D.
Gainesville, FL

Ralph F. Shangraw, Ph.D.
Baltimore, MD

Albert L. Sheffer, M.D.
Boston, MA

Eli Shefter, Ph.D
South San Francisco, CA

Eric B. Sheinin, Ph.D.
Rockville, MD

Jane C. Sheridan, Ph.D.
(1985–1988)
Nutley, NJ

Edward B. Silberstein, M.D.
Cincinnati, OH

Joseph E. Sinsheimer, Ph.D.
Ann Arbor, MI

Marilyn Dix Smith, Ph.D.
Stony Point, NY

Robert V. Smith, Ph.D.
Pullman, WA

E. John Staba, Ph.D.
Minneapolis, MN

Robert S. Stern, M.D.
Boston, MA

USP Advisory Panels 1985–1990

Members who serve as Chairmen are listed first.

The information presented in this text represents an ongoing review of the drugs contained herein and represents a consensus of various viewpoints expressed. The individuals listed below are currently on the USP Advisory Panels and have contributed to the development of the 1989 USP DI data base. Such listing does not imply that these individuals have reviewed all of the material in this text or that they individually agree with all statements contained herein.

Panel on Anesthesiology
Walter L. Way, M.D., San Francisco, CA; Frederic Berry, M.D., Charlottesville, VA; Roy Cronnelly, M.D., Ph.D., Somerset, CA; Dennis Mangano, M.D., Ph.D., San Francisco, CA; W. Jerry Merrell, M.D., Gainesville, FL; Carl Rosow, M.D., Ph.D., Boston, MA; Bradley Smith, M.D., Nashville, TN; Paul White, M.D., Ph.D., St. Louis, MO

Panel on Biological Tests and Assays
Terry E. Munson, B.S., Fairfax, VA; Robert L. Amos, Indianapolis, IN; Janet C. Curry, New York, NY; Herbert N. Prince, Ph.D., Fairfield, NJ

Panel on Bulk Packaging
Garnet E. Peck, Ph.D., West Lafayette, IN; Terry Benney, Ph.D., Philadelphia, PA; Gregory Haines, Union, NJ; Gordon E. Mallett, Ph.D., Indianapolis, IN

Panel on Cardiovascular and Renal Drugs
Edward D. Frohlich, M.D., New Orleans, LA; Emmanuel L. Bravo, M.D., Cleveland, OH; James E. Doherty, M.D., Little Rock, AR; Garabed Eknoyan, M.D., Houston, TX; Ruth Eshleman, Ph.D., West Kingston, RI; Edward Genton, M.D., New Orleans, LA; Thomas M. Glenn, Ph.D., South San Francisco, CA; Norman K. Hollenberg, M.D., Ph.D., Boston, MA; John L. Juergens, M.D., Rochester, MN; Michael Lesch, M.D., Chicago, IL; Benjamin F. McGraw, Pharm.D., Kansas City, MO; Patrick A. McKee, M.D., Oklahoma City, OK; Bernard L. Mirkin, Ph.D., M.D., Minneapolis, MN; Burton E. Sobel, M.D., St. Louis, MO; W. David Watkins, M.D., Ph.D., Durham, NC

Panel on Clinical Immunology
Albert L. Sheffer, M.D., Boston, MA; John Baum, M.D., Rochester, NY; Jonathan S. Coblyn, M.D., Brookline, MA; Elliot F. Ellis, M.D., Buffalo, NY; Patricia A. Fraser, M.D., Boston, MA; Thomas Gilman, Pharm.D., Los Angeles, CA; Stephen R. Kaplan, M.D., Providence, RI; Sandra Koehler, Milwaukee, WI; Floyd Malveaux, M.D., Ph.D., Washington, DC; Edward B. Nelson, M.D., Ph.D.,

Houston, TX; Robert E. Reisman, M.D., Buffalo, NY; Daniel J. Stechschulte, M.D., Kansas City, KS; Martin D. Valentine, M.D., Baltimore, MD

Panel on Consumer Interest
James Rankin, B.S., Santa Fe, NM; Judith Brown, B.A., Washington, DC; Jose Camacho, Austin, TX; Margaret A. Charters, Ph.D., Syracuse, NY; Jennifer Cross, San Francisco, CA; Gabriel Daniel, Washington, DC; John Forbes, Rio Piedras, PR; Jerome Halperin, Edison, NJ; Anita M. LeValdo, Window Rock, AZ; Janice Lieberman, Buffalo, NY; Esther Peterson, Washington, DC; Ruth Richards, M.A., M.P.H., Los Angeles, CA; T. Donald Rucker, Ph.D., Chicago, IL; Gordon Schiff, M.D., Chicago, IL

Panel on Dentistry
Sebastian G. Ciancio, D.D.S., Buffalo, NY; Donald F. Adams, D.D.S., Portland, OR; Karen Baker, M.S., Iowa City, IA; Priscilla C. Bourgault, Ph.D., Maywood, IL; Frederick A. Curro, D.M.D., Ph.D., Jersey City, NJ; Phyllis Eliasberg, Boston, MA; Tommy W. Gage, D.D.S., Ph.D., Dallas, TX; Stephen F. Goodman, D.D.S., New York, NY; Zack Kasloff, D.D.S., Winnipeg, Manitoba, Canada; Joseph Margarone, D.D.S., Buffalo, NY; Michael Newman, D.D.S., Los Angeles, CA; James W. Smudski, D.M.D., Ph.D., Pittsburgh, PA; Clarence L. Trummel, D.D.S., Ph.D., Farmington, CT; Raymond P. White, Jr., D.D.S., Ph.D., Chapel Hill, NC

Panel on Dermatology
Robert S. Stern, M.D., Boston, MA; Richard D. Baughman, M.D., Hanover, NH; Michael Bigby, M.D., Brookline, MA; Henry Jolly, M.D., New Orleans, LA; W. Stuart Maddin, M.D., F.R.C.P., Vancouver, British Columbia, Canada; Milton Orkin, M.D., Minneapolis, MN; Edgar Benton Smith, M.D., Galveston, TX; John Strauss, M.D., Iowa City, IA; Dennis West, M.S., Chicago, IL; Gail Zimmerman, B.A., Portland, OR

Panel on Diagnostic Agents—Nonradioactive
Harry W. Fischer, M.D., Rochester, NY; James A. Nelson, M.D., Seattle, WA; Robert L. Siegle, M.D., San Antonio, TX; Jovitas Skucas, M.D., Rochester, NY; William M. Thompson, M.D., Minneapolis, MN; Gerald L. Wolf, Ph.D., M.D., Pittsburgh, PA

Panel on Endocrinology
Dean H. Lockwood, M.D., Rochester, NY; Louis V. Avioli, M.D., St. Louis, MO; Edwin D. Bransome, Jr., M.D., Augusta, GA; P. Reed Larsen, M.D., Boston, MA; Marvin E. Levin, M.D., St. Louis, MO; Marvin M. Lipman, M.D., Mt. Vernon, NY; Walter J. Meyer, III., M.D., Galveston, TX; Rita Nemchik, R.N., M.S., Philadelphia, PA; Maria New, M.D., New York, NY; John A Owen, M.D., Charlottesville, VA; Robert W. Rebar, M.D., Cincinnati, OH; Thomas H. Wiser, Pharm.D., Buies Creek, NC

Panel on In-vitro Toxicity Testing

Robert V. Petersen, Ph.D., Salt Lake City, UT; Scott A. Burton, Ph.D., St. Paul, MN; Thomas F. Genova, Ph.D., Somerville, NJ; Alan Goldberg, Ph.D., Baltimore, MD; Richard D. Henry, Philadelphia, PA; Barbara H. Keech, Vienna, VA; Tibor Matula, Ph.D., Ottawa, Ont., Canada; Jerry Nelson, Ph.D., Salt Lake City, UT; Daniel L. Prince, Ph.D., Fairfield, NJ; Thomas D. Sabourin, Ph.D., Columbus, OH; Adelbert L. Stagg, Ph.D., Research Triangle Park, NC; D. M. Stark, D.V.M., Ph.D., New York, NY; Richard F. Wallin, D.V.M., Ph.D., Northwood, OH

Panel on Moisture Specifications

George Zografi, Ph.D., Madison, WI; R. Gary Hollenbeck, Ph.D., Baltimore, MD; Sharon Laughlin, Ph.D., Groton, CT; Mikal J. Pikal, Ph.D., Indianapolis, IN; Joseph B. Schwartz, Ph.D., Philadelphia, PA; Lynn Van Campen, Ph.D., Ridgefield, CT

Panel on Neurological and Psychiatric Disease

Burton J. Goldstein, M.D., F.A.C.P., Miami, FL; Alex A. Cardoni, M.S., Hartford, CT; James C. Cloyd, Pharm.D., Minneapolis, MN; N. Michael Davis, M.S., Miami, FL; Richard Dorsey, M.D., Newport Beach, CA; Larry Ereshefsky, Pharm.D., San Antonio, TX; W. Edwin Fann, M.D., Houston, TX; Kathleen M. Foley, M.D., New York, NY; Tracy R. Gordy, M.D., Austin, TX; I.K. Ho, Ph.D., Jackson, MS; Chung Y. Hsu, M.D., Ph.D., Charleston, SC; J. Kiffin Penry, M.D., Winston-Salem, NC; Michael A. Taylor, M.D., North Chicago, IL; Sister Ann Walton, St. Paul, MN; Michael Weintraub, M.D., Rochester, NY; Stanley van den Noort, M.D., Irvine, CA

Panel on Nursing Practice

Faye Abdellah, R.N., Ed.D., Sc.D., Rockville, MD; Col. Naldean Borg, Olympia, WA; Mecca S. Cranley, R.N., Ph.D., Madison, WI; Barbara A. Durand, R.N.C., Ed.D., F.A.A.N., Chicago, IL; Hector Hugo Gonzales, R.N., Ph.D., San Antonio, TX; Laurie Martin Gunter, Ph.D., R.N., F.A.A.N., Seattle, WA; Gloria S. Hope, R.N., Ph.D., Washington, DC; Jean Marshall, B.A., R.N., Lakewood, NJ; Ida M. Martinson, R.N., Ph.D., San Francisco, CA; Loretta Nowakowski, R.N., Ph.D., New Castle, PA; Carol P. Patton, R.N., Ph.D., J.D., Ann Arbor, MI; Sharon S. Rising, R.N., C.N.M., Cheshire, CT; Franklin A. Shaffer, R.N., Ed.D., New York, NY; Margaret D. Sovie, R.N., Ph.D., Philadelpha, PA; Una Beth Westfall, R.N., Seattle, WA

Panel on Nutrition and Electrolytes

Robert D. Lindeman, M.D., Washington, DC; William O. Berndt, Ph.D., Omaha, NE; Steven B. Heymsfield, M.D., New York, NY; Bonnie Liebman, M.S., Washington, DC; Timothy Lipman, M.D., Washington, DC; Sudesh K. Mahajan, M.D., Allen Park, MI; David J. Martin, Pharm.D., Atlanta, GA; Robert M. Russell, M.D., Boston,

Washington, D.C.; W. Manford Gooch, III, M.D., Salt Lake City, UT; Ralph E. Kauffman, M.D., Detroit, MI; Joan M. Korth-Bradley, Pharm.D., Edmonton, Alberta, Canada; Robert H. Levin, Pharm.D., San Francisco, CA; Paul A. Palmisano, M.D., Birmingham, AL; Albert W. Pruitt, M.D., Augusta, GA; Philip D. Walson, M.D., Columbus, OH; Sumner J. Yaffe, M.D., Bethesda, MD

Panel on Pharmacy Practice
William F. Appel, D.Sc., Minneapolis, MN; Henry Cade, B.S., Chicago, IL; Herbert S. Carlin, D.Sc., Chappaqua, NY; Olya Duzey, M.S., Reed City, MI; Frances Hall Grogan, B.S., Wickliffe, KY; Ned Heltzer, M.S., Santa Fe, NM; James E. Hosch, B.S., Kansas City, KS; Patricia A. Kramer, B.S., Bismarck, ND; Shirley P. McKee, B.S., Houston, TX; Thomas P. Reinders, Pharm.D., Richmond, VA; Lorie G. Rice, B.A., M.P.H., Sacramento, CA; Al Sebok, B.S., Twinsburg, OH; Stephen M. Sleight, M.S., Bay Pines, FL; William E. Smith, Pharm.D., M.P.H., Long Beach, CA; Thomas C. Snader, Pharm.D., Furlong, PA; J. Richard Wuest, Pharm.D., Cincinnati, OH

Panel on Radiopharmaceuticals
Edward B. Silberstein, M.D., Cincinnati, OH; Neil M. Abel, M.B.A., M.S., Rockville, MD; William H. Briner, Capt., B.S., Durham, NC; Henry Chilton, Pharm.D., Winston-Salem, NC; Jan M. Ellerhorst-Ryan, R.N., M.S.N., C.S., Cincinnati, OH; Richard Holmes, M.D., Columbia, MO; William Kaplan, M.D., Boston, MA; David L. Laven, C.R.Ph., F.A.S.C.P., Bay Pines, FL; Merle K. Loken, M.D., Ph.D., Minneapolis, MN; Norman L. McElroy, M.A., Washington, DC; William B. Nelp, M.D., Seattle, WA; Buck A. Rhodes, Ph.D., Albuquerque, NM; Barry A. Siegel, M.D., St. Louis, MO; Guy Simmons, Ph.D., Lexington, KY; Dennis P. Swanson, R.Ph., M.S., Detroit, MI; David A. Weber, Ph.D., Upton, NY; Henry N. Wellman, M.D., Indianapolis, IN

Panel on Radiopharmaceuticals Standards
William H. Briner, Capt., B.S., Durham, NC; Jacqueline M. Calhoun, Gaithersburg, MD; Paul Early, Cleveland, OH

Panel on Sterility and Microbial Attributes
Murray S. Cooper, Ph.D., Islamarada, FL; Frank W. Adair, Ph.D., Summit, NJ; William C. Alegnani, Ph.D., Rochester, MI; R. Michael Enzinger, Ph.D., Kalamazoo, MI; Henry Jarocha, R.Ph., Rochester, NJ; Eugene A. Timm, Ph.D., Rochester, MI; C. Searle Wadley, North Chicago, IL

Panel on Sterilization Indicators
Virginia C. Chamberlain, Silver Spring, MD; Henry L. Avallone, North Brunswick, NJ; David Bekus, Somerville, NJ; Robert Berube, Ph.D., St. Paul, MN; Frank B. Engley, Jr., Ph.D., Columbia, MO; Gary S. Graham, Ph.D., Erie, PA; Lois A. Jones, Research Triangle

Park, NC; Karl Kereluk, Ph.D. (deceased), Rouses Point, NY; Ruth B. Kundsin, Sc.D., Boston, MA; Patrick McCormick, Ph.D., Rochester, NY; Gregg A. Mosley, Belgrade, MT; Theron E. Odlaug, Ph.D., Elkhart, IN; Gordon S. Oxborrow, Minneapolis, MN

Panel on Surgical Drugs and Devices
James W. Pate, M.D., Memphis, TN; C. Andrew Bassett, M.D., New York, NY; Terry Baumann, Pharm.D., Detroit, MI; Peter J. Fabri, M.D., Tampa, FL; Susan Bartlett Foote, J.D., Berkeley, CA; Jack Hirsh, M.D., Hamilton, Ontario, Canada; Larry R. Pilot, Esq., Washington, DC; Lary A. Robinson, M.D., Omaha, NE; H. Harlan Stone, M.D., Cleveland, OH; Clark Watts, M.D., Columbia, MO

Panel on Urology
Saul Boyarsky, M.D., St. Louis, MO; John Belis, M.D., Hershey, PA; Michael Boileau, M.D., Bend, OR; Culley C. Carson, M.D., Durham, NC; Warren Heston, Ph.D., New York, NY; Mark V. Jarowenko, M.D., Hershey, PA, Marguerite Lippert, M.D., Charlottesville, VA; Penelope A. Longhurst, Ph.D., Philadelphia, PA; Michael G. Mawhinney, Ph.D., Morgantown, WV; Harris Nagler, M.D., New York, NY; Randall H. Rowland, M.D., Ph.D., Indianapolis, IN; J. Patrick Spirnak, M.D., Cleveland, OH; William F. Tarry, M.D., Morgantown, WV; Alan J. Wein, M.D., Philadelphia, PA; Robert Weiss, M.D., New Haven, CT

Panel on Veterinary Medicine
Lloyd E. Davis, D.V.M., Ph.D., Urbana, IL; Arthur L. Aronson, D.V.M., Ph.D., Raleigh, NC; Nicholas H. Booth, D.V.M., Ph.D., Jacksonville, FL; Gordon L. Coppoc, D.V.M., Ph.D., West Lafayette, IN; Sidney A. Ewing, D.V.M., Ph.D., Stillwater, OK; Stuart D. Forney, M.S., Fort Collins, CO; Diane K. Gerken, D.V.M., Ph.D., Columbus, OH; William G. Huber, D.V.M., Blacksburg, VA; William L. Jenkins, D.V.M., Ph.D., Baton Rouge, LA; Robert W. Phillips, D.V.M., Ph.D., Fort Collins, CO; Thomas E. Powers, D.V.M., Ph.D., Columbus, OH; Charles R. Short, D.V.M., Ph.D., Baton Rouge, LA; Richard H. Teske, D.V.M., Rockville, MD; Jeffrey R. Wilcke, D.V.M., M.S., Blacksburg, VA

Headquarters Staff

DRUG INFORMATION DIVISION

Keith W. Johnson, *Director, Research and Development*

Assistant Director:
Georgie M. Cathey

Senior Pharmacy Associates:
Nancy Lee Dashiell
Esther Klein

Pharmacy Associates:
Debra Edwards
Wanda J. Janicki
Angela Méndez Mayo (Spanish Publications Coordinator)
Carol A. Pamer

Pharmacy Consultants:
Sandra Lee Boyer
Gordon K. Wurster

Publications Development:
Diana M. Blais (Coordinator)
Dorothy Raymond

Medical Information Specialist:
Martha A. D. Wollam

Research Assistants:
Eric M. Orr
Catherine E. Szabo

Editorial Consultant:
John Morris

Office Staff:
Mayra Martinez
Jaime Ramirez

Student Interns/Fellows:
Eugenie Brown (University of Texas)
Daniel C. Loper (University of Georgia)
Kimberly Werner (University of Illinois)

PUBLICATION SERVICES

Patricia H. Morgenstern, *Director*
Mary C. Griffiths (Ret.)

Managing Editor, USP DI:
A. V. Precup

Editorial Associates, USP DI:
Carol M. Griffin
Elizabeth C. Horowitz
Ellen R. Loeb
Marianne T. Martin

Typesetters:
Lori E. Foster (Supervisor)
Deborah R. Connelly
Lauren Taylor Davis
Myra Spencer

Typesetting Systems Coordinator:
Jean E. Dale

Graphics Coordinator:
Gail M. Oring

Also Contributing: Joan Goldenberg, Judy Jason, Diana Madden, and Andrea Newsham Smith, Proofreaders; Tia Calomeris and Susan Messera, Graphics.

Managing Editor, USP-NF:
Sandra Boynton

Editorial Associates, USP-NF:
Jesusa D. Cordova
Ellen Elovitz
Carolyn A. Fleeger
Suzanne Lassandro
Melissa Smith

About the National High Blood Pressure Education Program

Since 1972, federal, state, and community programs have been working together on a cooperative program to control high blood pressure. This comprehensive effort, the National High Blood Pressure Education Program (NHBPEP), has focused on increasing public and professional awareness about this serious health problem. The educational goal of all Program participants has been to reduce high blood pressure–related death and disability through improved detection and treatment efforts.

As an educational program, the NHBPEP encourages both acceptance and application of existing knowledge and techniques. Program participants have assumed an active role in addressing the attitudes, beliefs, and practices of professionals, patients, community projects, and government agencies, as well as the general public.

The magnitude and complexity of high blood pressure as a public health problem has dictated the Program's comprehensive strategy: to mobilize, educate, and coordinate the resources and energies of all interested government and private sector groups. Under the leadership of the National Heart, Lung, and Blood Institute (NHLBI), the joint national effort includes numerous Federal agencies, virtually all state health departments, and more than 150 private sector organizations, such as professional societies, voluntary health associations, certifying and accrediting bodies, pharmaceutical companies, labor and management groups, and insurance companies. Hundreds of community efforts are also allied with the Program and are involved in every facet of high blood pressure control.

The National Program follows a consensus-building process to identify major issues and develop strategies. As part of this consensus-building approach, representatives from more than 32 key NHBPEP participant groups work together on the National High Blood Pressure Coordinating Committee to offer mutual support and guidance for Program strategies. This multi-disciplinary committee, currently chaired by the director of the NHLBI, defines national priorities, examines critical issues, considers future opportunities, and facilitates collaboration among the many organizations involved in control.

The NHBPEP's examination of major high blood pressure control issues includes a range of perspectives: the appropriate roles of health care professionals; the most effective treatment practices in medical management; high blood pressure control at the worksite; the needs of rural communities; high blood pressure in elderly people; the relationship of diet and high blood pressure; the safety and accuracy of automatic blood pressure measurement devices; and others.

About
High
Blood
Pressure

About High Blood Pressure

What is blood pressure?

When your heart beats, it pumps blood through your blood vessels. The force of the blood that is pumped out then pushes against the walls of these vessels and creates the force known as blood pressure. In fact, blood pressure is the force that keeps blood moving through the vessels.

Blood pressure is expressed in terms of millimeters of mercury (mm Hg) and consists of two values. For example, normal blood pressure for an adult is usually around 120/80 mm Hg. The upper (first) value is called systolic blood pressure. It describes the force that occurs when the heart pumps, pushing blood out into the arteries. The lower (second) value is called diastolic blood pressure. It describes the pressure inside the blood vessels when the heart relaxes.

Blood pressure may vary even when it is normal. It is usually lowest when you are asleep, but it may increase if you are excited or nervous or when you are exercising. It may also be increased by a sudden injury or when you smoke a cigarette or drink coffee. However, these are only temporary increases and your blood pressure goes back down to its usual level after a short time.

What is high blood pressure?

High blood pressure is an abnormally elevated amount of pressure of the blood against the blood vessels. This happens if your vessels clamp down or tighten, making it harder for the blood to flow and causing your blood pressure to rise in order to overcome the resistance created by the constriction of the blood vessels.

Hypertension is the medical term for high blood pressure. It *does not* refer to nervous tension. *Primary* or *essential* hypertension refers to a type of high blood pressure for which the exact cause is unknown, although it tends to run in families. The term essential comes from an old medical misunderstanding and should not be understood to mean that the elevated pressure is necessary.

From now on , when the term "high blood pressure" is used in this book, it will refer to primary or essential hypertension.

Most doctors define hypertension as a diastolic pressure of greater than 90 mm Hg, usually associated with a systolic pressure of greater than 140 mm Hg. When blood pressure is only slightly elevated, the condition is called "mild hypertension." Even mild hypertension, if left untreated, can be serious.

What causes high blood pressure?

High blood pressure, contrary to popular belief, is not caused by tension or nervousness, although too much emotional upset may elevate it. Essential hypertension has no known cause and is the type that occurs in approximately 85 percent of patients having high blood pressure. For the remaining 15 percent, different causes may be responsible for the elevated blood pressure. For example, some cases may be caused by a tumor or may be the result of kidney disease or narrowing of one of the blood vessels to the kidney, disease of the adrenal gland, or other hormonal abnormalities.

Although the exact cause of essential hypertension is unknown, there are certain personal factors that may identify a person to be more likely to develop hypertension. In many people, a combination of these factors may be involved. For example, the frequency of occurrence of hypertension is generally greater in men, in blacks, in persons over 50 years of age, and in those who have a family history of hypertension. In addition, some people are overly sensitive to sodium (salt) and may be more likely to develop or aggravate hypertension because of this.

How is high blood pressure detected?

Hypertension usually does not produce any noticeable signs of the disease until it has been present for a long time. Your doctor may discover that you have it by taking a routine blood pressure measurement before symptoms develop. However, one high measurement does not necessarily mean that you have high blood pressure. It could be due to emotional upset, anger, or recent exercise. Several measurements that are consistently high when you are lying down, sitting, and standing, however, may mean that you have hypertension.

Why does high blood pressure need to be treated?

Most doctors now recommend treatment of high blood pressure, even when it is not very much above normal. High blood pressure adds to the workload of the heart and arteries. If it continues for a long time, the heart and arteries may not function properly. This can damage the blood vessels of the brain, heart, and kidneys, resulting in a stroke, heart failure, or kidney failure. Hypertension is also a major risk factor underlying heart attacks. These problems may be less likely to occur if blood pressure is controlled.

The amount of damage that hypertension causes is related to how high the blood pressure is and how long it has been elevated. Therefore, it is best to treat hypertension early, before damage occurs or gets worse.

Myths About High Blood Pressure

There are some common misconceptions about high blood pressure:

Myth: If I feel well, then my blood pressure must be normal.

In most people, there are no symptoms of hypertension; it is detected through blood pressure measurements.

Myth: Only tense, anxious people get high blood pressure.

Anyone can have high blood pressure and the cause may not be known. There are approximately 58 million people in the United States who have high blood pressure. While emotional upset will raise your blood pressure temporarily, this does not cause the condition; even very calm, relaxed people can develop high blood pressure.

Myth: High blood pressure can be treated with tranquilizers.

Tranquilizers generally are *not* useful in treating hypertension since it is not caused by tension; they do not lower blood pressure. What *is* useful is a program of medication, and possibly diet, exercise, and stress reduction, that you and your doctor will work out together.

Myth: High blood pressure is a disease of old age.

People of *all* ages can develop high blood pressure, although people over 50 years of age are more likely to have it. Even children can have hypertension; however, the cause is often different in children than in adults.

Myth: Essential high blood pressure can be cured.

Essential hypertension is a condition that usually requires *lifelong* treatment; it can be controlled, but it cannot be cured. However, some other types of hypertension can be cured.

Myth: High blood pressure significantly restricts my life.

This should not be true. With your participation in the planning and carrying out of your treatment, you can lead a normal life; however, early, proper, and continued treatment is necessary to prevent the damage that untreated blood pressure can cause.

Making the Decision to Treat High Blood Pressure

Treatment may involve any or all of the following:

Diet—Your doctor may want you to follow a diet that is low in sodium and fats; in addition, if you are overweight, a diet prescribed by your doctor and dietitian that will help you lose weight may help bring your blood pressure under control. It may also reduce the amount of antihypertensive medicines that you must take if they are still required.

Exercise—This may help you to lose weight and be healthier; however, always check with your doctor before starting a new exercise program, especially if you are over 40 years of age, since some forms of exercise are better than others for different patients.

Smoking avoidance—Smoking greatly increases the risks of heart and blood vessel disease associated with hypertension and should be avoided.

Stress reduction—Stress reduction alone will probably not lower your blood pressure, but it may help the other methods of treatment to be more effective.

Medication—If treatment without medication involving the above-mentioned changes in lifestyle is not sufficient, drug therapy may be added. Since there are many different kinds of high blood pressure medicine, your doctor will determine which is the best for your particular condition.

Before starting treatment for your high blood pressure, there is an important decision that you must make:

You must decide whether you are willing to commit yourself to getting your high blood pressure under control. Whether it is controlled or not depends on you. Your doctor can prescribe medicine and suggest treatment. Only you can decide to follow through.

Treating your hypertension may necessitate some changes in your lifestyle which will probably last the rest of your life. By learning about your condition and becoming a partner with your doctor in your treatment, *you can be the decision-maker in your own care.*

Your chances of living an active, healthy life are good if you treat your high blood pressure wisely.

Before you make any decision, there are several important things that you should remember:

Essential hypertension can be controlled but it cannot be cured. Unfortunately, essential hypertension can only be controlled, not cured, since no one really knows what causes it. If you stop your treatment when your blood pressure improves, it will go up again. Your blood pressure will be monitored and you will probably have to follow some kind of treatment all your life.

Most people with high blood pressure do not have any symptoms. Most individuals do not have any noticeable symptoms of the high blood pressure until after it has damaged the blood vessels and the heart.

The only way to know is by having your blood pressure measured.

Treatment of high blood pressure is a lifelong prospect. Because high blood pressure often has no symptoms, you may be tempted to stop taking your medicine or go off your nondrug treatment. After all, you feel fine, and your medicine may cause some uncomfortable side effects or be inconvenient to take or your nondrug treatment may be difficult to follow. However, *if you stop your treatment, your blood pressure will not be controlled* and you run the increased risk of stroke, heart failure, heart attack, or kidney failure.

You must become a partner in your treatment. Your doctor alone cannot bring your blood pressure under control. With your help and participation, it will be easier for both of you, working as a team, to control your blood pressure.

Treating high blood pressure successfully requires that you make some changes in your lifestyle. You may have to make some changes in your diet and daily routine. Controlling your weight and cutting down on sodium or cholesterol may help control your blood pressure. Medication-taking should be tailored to your daily schedule so it will become a natural habit.

If taking medication, you may notice some side effects: In addition to their helpful effects, most medicines may have some side effects, some of which are serious while others are only bothersome. If you experience side effects, you and your doctor can decide together whether to change the dose of the medicine or to switch to another medicine. However, there may be some side effects that cannot be avoided.

Each patient is different and medicine may not act the same for everyone. If one medicine does not work well enough, your doctor may try another. Just because you start taking one medicine does not mean you will always take that same medicine.

Never change the dose of your medicine or stop taking it or change your nondrug treatment without discussing it with your doctor. You must decide *together* on the best thing to do.

Dietary Treatment of High Blood Pressure

Cutting down on salt

Sodium (most commonly thought of as table salt or sodium chloride) is important in maintaining proper levels of fluid in your body. Other forms of sodium in our diet may be included in any number of salts (e.g., sodium ascorbate, sodium bicarbonate, sodium citrate, sodium glutamate) used to process and preserve canned, frozen, and processed foods. Too much sodium has been linked with hypertension, especially in people who are overly sensitive to it. You need only 200 mg of sodium a day (with no more than 3300 mg generally recommended), but many adults in North America take in 10,000–15,000 mg daily, mostly from food. Sodium is also present in certain sweeteners (e.g., sodium saccharin), antacids (e.g., sodium bicarbonate), and medicines (e.g., sodium pentobarbital).

Your doctor may ask you to reduce the amount of sodium in your diet. This will generally help reduce the amount of medicine you need to take to control your hypertension.

In general, highly processed or convenience foods contain large amounts of sodium, while fresh fruits and vegetables are low in sodium. Because salt is used in many ways in food processing, it often cannot be tasted and therefore may appear as "hidden" salt.

Many manufacturers are now listing on the label the amount of sodium contained in foods or medicines. Look for the number of mg of sodium or check the list of ingredients for substances with "sodium" in their names. If these substances appear early on in the ingredient list, it may mean that the item is high in sodium.

Remember that salt is an acquired taste. We learn to like salt and we can learn to like less of it. By cutting down on salt gradually, and using other spices instead, many people find that they prefer the taste of foods without salt added.

Cutting down on fats

In addition to increasing the risk of hardening of the arteries (atherosclerosis), heart disease (coronary artery disease), heart attacks, and strokes, a high cholesterol level in the blood increases the risks associated with hypertension. In fact, it may be the narrowing and stiffening of the arteries due to fat buildup that tends to drive blood pressure up.

Cutting down on fat in the diet will be beneficial in several ways. It will help reduce the risk of heart disease, strokes, and possibly hypertension. It will also help in weight control.

Weight control

Obesity is also a known risk factor in hypertension. Many people with only mild hypertension find that they can bring their blood pressure down merely by controlling their weight. However, blood pressure stays down only as long as the weight stays down.

It is a good idea to check with your doctor and dietitian before starting a reducing diet. Weight loss should be gradual and based on a nutritionally sound diet so that healthy eating habits can be maintained for life.

Alcohol

Some doctors believe that drinking moderate amounts of alcohol (1 to 2 ounces a day) may actually help reduce the risk of hypertension. However, while it is true that alcohol may reduce blood pressure in the short run, chronic excessive use (more than 2 ounces a day) has actually been found to lead to hypertension and possibly other diseases.

Moderation is the key. Discuss with your doctor how much alcohol you can drink.

The Role of Smoking

Smoking is associated with an increased risk of cardiovascular disease, including heart attacks and strokes. Hypertension also increases the risk of heart and blood vessel disease and the combination with smoking causes the risk to be much greater. The risk is only slightly less with cigars and pipes than with cigarettes. Therefore, it is very important to avoid smoking. Although it will not lower blood pressure, it will help reduce the risks associated with hypertension. It will also reduce other risks associated with smoking, such as lung cancer, bronchitis, and emphysema.

Reducing Stress to Reduce Blood Pressure

As discussed earlier, hypertension is not a type of emotional tension and it is not caused by tension or nervousness. Even relaxed people can have hypertension. However, stressful situations do tend to temporarily increase blood pressure and chronic stress may aggravate or increase the risk of hypertension.

Reducing stress in your life will not lower your blood pressure to normal, but along with other treatments (medication and diet), it may help control it.

Drug Treatment of High Blood Pressure

How do high blood pressure medicines work?

There are several different kinds of antihypertensive medicines. Although their actions may be different, all help to lower blood pressure.

- Diuretics or "water pills"—Help reduce the amount of salt and water in the body by increasing the flow of urine. Examples are thiazide diuretics, loop diuretics, and potassium-sparing diuretics.

- Beta-adrenergic blocking agents—Help reduce the workload of the heart by affecting the response to some nerve impulses in the heart and blood vessels. Examples are acebutolol, atenolol, carteolol, labetalol, metoprolol, nadolol, penbutolol, pindolol, propranolol, and timolol.

- Calcium channel blocking agents—Affect the movement of calcium into the cells of the heart and blood vessels. As a result, they relax the blood vessels and reduce the workload of the heart. Examples are diltiazem, nifedipine, and verapamil.

- Medicines that act directly on blood vessels— Relax blood vessels so that blood passes through them more easily. Examples are hydralazine and minoxidil.

- Medicines that act on the nervous system—
Relax blood vessels by controlling nerve impulses
along certain nerve pathways. Examples are
clonidine, guanabenz, guanadrel, guanethidine,
methyldopa, pargyline, prazosin, rauwolfia
alkaloids, and terazosin.

- Angiotensin-converting enzyme (ACE)
inhibitors—Block an enzyme in the blood that
causes blood vessels to tighten and as a result,
relax blood vessels. Examples are captopril,
enalapril, and lisinopril.

How many medicines will I have to take?

Many patients, especially those with mild
hypertension, need to take only one medicine.
However, others may require two or more to bring
their blood pressure under control. In these cases, a
diuretic usually will be given along with an
antihypertensive that relaxes blood vessels. Your doctor
may have to try different medicines at different
dosages until the combination that works best for you
and causes you the least side effects is found. Many
doctors follow what is called a "stepped-care program"
for treatment of hypertension. This involves starting
with one kind of medicine, adjusting the dose, and
then adding or changing to other medicines in a
certain order, if and when they are needed. Your
doctor may also try to reduce drug dosages after your
blood pressure is controlled.

How can I fit medication-taking into my life?

**Plan the times that you take your medicine into
your normal daily routine so that you develop a natural
habit.** You can take your medicine before you brush
your teeth, wash your face, eat breakfast or other
meals, shave, watch television, or anything else that
you do every day. Associating taking your medicine

with other things you do will also help you remember to take it. Pick out anything that works for *you*. However, some medicines have effects that may be particularly inconvenient at certain times of the day, such as drowsiness or frequent urination. Also, some antihypertensives should be taken on an empty stomach. You and your doctor and pharmacist can work out the best time of day for you to take your medicine so that these effects will interfere with your life as little as possible.

Your doctor may suggest that you take your own blood pressure measurements. By measuring your own blood pressure, you can help manage your treatment program and watch your progress in bringing it under control.

Your doctor or nurse can teach you the proper way and the best time to take a blood pressure measurement. Remember that your blood pressure may be slightly different at different times of day, or if you are sick or have a fever. Check with your doctor if you are concerned about a change in your blood pressure. Also, your blood pressure measurement equipment should be periodically checked to ensure that it is taking accurate measurements.

Keep all of your doctor's appointments. Even if you feel well, it is important that your doctor check your progress at periodic intervals. This also gives you a chance to ask any questions you may have.

If you can't make it to your appointment, let your doctor know and make a new appointment for as soon as is convenient for you.

Once your blood pressure is under control, visits to the doctor will become less frequent.

Ask questions. Knowing as much as possible about your condition and its treatment will help you in bringing it under control.

Write down questions when you think of them so that you will remember to ask your doctor at your next visit. Don't be afraid to ask questions. If something is of special concern to you, call your doctor, nurse, dietitian, or pharmacist. They are interested in your care and want to know your feelings, concerns, fears, and questions. The best way to help is to be informed about your condition.

Make a medication calendar. This will help you to keep track of your own treatment and to remember to take your medicine. Instructions for keeping such a calendar and samples that you can clip and use can be found in the back of this book.

Keep a diary to record your progress. The clip-out wallet diaries in this book will allow you to keep your own record of your blood pressure measurements, your doctor's appointments, and special instructions about medicine prescribed for you.

Be a partner with your doctor, nurse, dietitian, and pharmacist. Getting your blood pressure under control requires close teamwork, and you are a key member of the team. Make the decision to follow your treatment and work with your doctor, nurse, dietitian, and pharmacist to make it as successful as possible.

Enlist your family's or friends' help. Remember, they need you and want you to have the longest, healthiest life possible. They can help you remember to take your medicine, follow your diet, or check your blood pressure. Have them read this book so they can understand your condition. Put *them* on your team, too.

What should I know about my medicines?

Whenever you start taking a new medicine, you should ask:

> • When should I take the medicine? You need to know how often it should be taken, at what

time(s) of day, or with food or on an empty stomach.

- How much medicine should I take at one time?

- What should I do if I miss a dose?

- What are the common side effects of the medicine? Your doctor will tell you when the prescription is written what side effects there are, if any, and what to do about them. You can also read about your medicines in this book or ask your pharmacist.

- How can I minimize these side effects?

- Can I take other medicines while I take this high blood pressure medicine? Remember that your doctor should be told about all medicines you take, even over-the-counter (nonprescription) medicines such as aspirin, antacids, laxatives, and cold medicines.

- Can my diet affect the way the medicine works?

- What restrictions, if any, should I be aware of while I take this medicine? These might include avoidance of or caution while driving or operating hazardous machinery, or wearing a medication identification bracelet.

- Can this medicine be taken while I am pregnant or if I am breast-feeding?

- When should I seek help if problems arise?

- How much will this medicine cost?

- Can this prescription be written as a generic name instead of a brand name to save money?

- How long will the medicine remain potent after I purchase it?

For More Information About High Blood Pressure

If you want to learn more about high blood pressure, check with your doctor, nurse, and pharmacist. You can also obtain information from the following sources. You may find them in your local area.

- State and local public health departments
- American and state Heart Associations
- National and state Kidney Foundations
- Red Cross Chapters
- American Dietetic Association
- American Hospital Association
- Local hospitals or clinics (contact patient education coordinator)

Many books about health, high blood pressure, and medicines can be found in your local library or bookstore. Your community may also have a special blood pressure program. In addition, the National High Blood Pressure Information Center makes available free of charge many consumer and patient materials. An order form with titles and descriptions can be found as an appendix to this book or write to:

National High Blood Pressure Information Center
120/80 National Institutes of Health
Bethesda, MD 20892

REMEMBER:

- It's *your* health and future that are at stake.
- Bringing your blood pressure under control is a challenge you cannot ignore.
- High blood pressure is a lifelong disease that can affect all of your body's important organs.
- Be an active partner in your treatment. By meeting this challenge, you can enjoy an active and healthy life.

General Information About Use of Medicines

General Information About Use of Medicines

Information about the proper use of medicines is of two types. One type is drug specific and applies to a certain medicine or group of medicines only. The other type is general in nature and applies to the use of any medicine.

The information that follows is general in nature. For your own safety, health, and well-being, however, it is important that you learn about the proper use of your specific medicines as well. You can get this information from your doctor, nurse, or pharmacist, or find it in the individual listings of this book.

Before Using Your Medicine

Before you use any medicine, your doctor, nurse, and pharmacist should be told:

—if you have ever had an allergic or unusual reaction to any medicine, food, or other substance, such as yellow dye or sulfites.

—if you are on a low-salt, low-sugar, or any other special diet. Most medicines contain more than their active ingredient, and many liquid medicines contain alcohol.

—**if you are pregnant or if you plan to become pregnant.** Certain medicines may cause birth defects or other problems in the unborn child. For other medicines, safe use during pregnancy has not been established. **The use of any medicine during pregnancy must be carefully considered.**

—**if you are breast-feeding.** Some medicines may pass into the breast milk and cause unwanted effects in the baby.

—**if you have any medical problems.**

—**if you are now taking or have taken any medicines in the past few weeks.** Don't forget over-the-counter (nonprescription) medicines such as aspirin, laxatives, and antacids.

Proper Use of Your Medicine

Take medicine exactly as directed, at the right time, and for the full length of time prescribed by your doctor. If you are using an over-the-counter (nonprescription) medicine, follow the directions on the label, unless otherwise directed by your doctor. If you feel that your medicine is not working for you, check with your doctor.

To avoid mistakes, do not take medicine in the dark. Always read the label before taking, noting especially the expiration date, if any, of the contents.

Child-proof caps on medicines for oral use have greatly decreased the number of accidental poisonings and are required by law. However, if there are no children in your home, and you find it hard to open such caps, you may ask your pharmacist for a regular, easier-to-open cap. He or she is authorized by law to furnish you with a regular cap if you request it.

Different medicines should never be mixed in one container. Always keep your medicine tightly capped in its original container, when not in use. Do not remove the label since directions for use and other special information appear there.

It is important to store your medicines properly. Guidelines for proper storage include:

- **Keep out of the reach of children.**

- Store away from heat and direct light.

- Do not store capsules or tablets in the bathroom, near the kitchen sink, or in other damp places. Heat or moisture may cause the medicine to break down.

- Keep liquid medicines from freezing.

- Do not store medicines in the refrigerator unless directed to do so.

- Do not keep outdated medicine or medicine no longer needed. Be sure that any discarded medicine is out of the reach of children.

Precautions While Using Your Medicine

Never give your medicine to anyone else. It has been prescribed for your personal medical problem and may not be the correct treatment for another person.

Don't take medicines that show even the slightest evidence of tampering or don't seem quite right. If you have any questions, check with your pharmacist.

Before having any kind of surgery (including dental surgery) or emergency treatment, tell the physician or dentist in charge about any medicine you are taking.

If you think you have taken an overdose of any medicine or if a child has taken a medicine by accident: Call your poison control center or your doctor or pharmacist at once. Keep those telephone numbers handy. Also, keep a bottle of Ipecac Syrup safely stored in your home in case you are told to cause vomiting. Read the directions on the label of Ipecac Syrup before using.

Side Effects of Your Medicine

Along with its intended effects, a medicine may cause some unwanted effects. Some of these side effects may need medical attention, while others may not. It is important for you to know what side effects may occur and what you should do if you notice signs of them. If you notice any unusual reactions or side effects that you were not told about, check with your doctor, nurse, or pharmacist.

Tips Against Tampering

Manufacturers of over-the-counter (OTC) medicines now package their products so that any evidence of tampering can be more readily noticed by the consumer. Manufacturers may use one or more different ways of packaging their products to make them tamper-resistant. These may include:

• Wrapping the dosage form and/or its container in a plastic film wrapper or bubble pack.

• Sealing each individual dosing unit in a foil, paper, or plastic pouch or in a blister or strip pack.

• Placing a shrink seal or band which fits tightly around the cap and container.

• Sealing the bottle mouth under the cap or the carton flaps with paper or foil seals or tape.

• Placing a breakable metal or plastic cap over the bottle opening.

General common sense suggestions to help you detect possible signs of tampering include the following:

• Take a few seconds to visually inspect the outer packaging of the drug product before you buy it and again as you open it. When you open the outer package after purchase, also check inner packaging features.

• If the medicine has a protective packaging feature, it should be intact. If it is not, do not buy the product or, if already purchased, return it to the store or manufacturer.

• Don't take medicines that show even the slightest evidence of tampering or that don't seem quite right.

• Never take medicines in the dark or in poor lighting. Look at the label and each dose of medicine *every time* you take a dose.

Additional Information

It is a good idea for you to learn both the generic and brand names of your medicine and even to write them down and keep them for future use.

Many prescriptions may not be refilled unless your pharmacist has first checked with your doctor. To save time, do not wait until you have run out of medicine before requesting a refill. This is especially important if you must take your medicine every day.

If you want more information about your medicines, ask your doctor, nurse, or pharmacist. Do not be embarrassed to ask questions about any medicine you are taking. To help you remember, it may be helpful to write down any questions you have and bring these questions with you on your next visit to your doctor or pharmacist.

About Your High Blood Pressure Medicines

The following information may provide general answers to some of your questions as well as suggestions for the correct use of your medicine. Medicines are complex, however, and may act differently on different people. If you feel that you need additional information about your medicine or its possible side effects, ask your doctor, nurse, or pharmacist. They are there to help you.

If any of the information causes you special concern, do not decide against taking any medicine prescribed for you without first checking with your doctor.

ANGIOTENSIN-CONVERTING ENZYME (ACE) INHIBITORS (Systemic)

This information applies to the following medicines:

Captopril (KAP-toe-pril)
Enalapril (e-NAL-a-pril)
Lisinopril (lyse-IN-oh-pril)

Some commonly used brand names are:

For Captopril
In the U.S. and Canada
     Capoten

For Enalapril
In the U.S. and Canada
     Vasotec

For Lisinopril†
In the U.S.
     Prinivil
     Zestril

---

†Not commercially available in Canada.

ACE inhibitors belong to the general class of medicines called antihypertensives. They are taken by mouth to treat high blood pressure.

High blood pressure adds to the workload of the heart and arteries. If it continues for a long time, the heart and arteries may not function properly. This can damage the blood vessels of the brain, heart, and kidneys, resulting in a stroke, heart failure, or kidney failure. High blood pressure may also increase the risk of heart attacks. These problems may be less likely to occur if blood pressure is controlled.

These medicines are also used to treat congestive heart failure.

The exact way that these medicines work is not known. They block an enzyme in the body that is necessary to produce a substance that causes blood vessels to tighten. As a result, they probably relax blood vessels. This lowers blood pressure and increases the supply of blood and oxygen to the heart.

These medicines are available only with your doctor's prescription.

Before Using This Medicine

To decide on the best treatment for your medical problem, your doctor should be told:

—if you have ever had any unusual or allergic reaction to captopril, enalapril, or lisinopril.

—if you are on a low-salt, low-sugar, or any other special diet, or if you are allergic to any substance, such as foods, sulfites or other preservatives, or dyes. Most medicines contain more than their active ingredient. Your doctor, nurse, or pharmacist can help you avoid products that may cause a problem.

—if you are **pregnant** or if you may become pregnant.

In humans, captopril has been reported to cause slowed growth of the fetus and difficulty in breathing and low blood pressure in the newborn. In addition, one case of a possible birth defect has been reported. Studies in rabbits and rats at doses up to 400 times the recommended human dose have shown that captopril causes an increase in deaths of the fetus and newborn. Also, captopril has caused deformed skulls in rabbits.

Studies with enalapril have not been done in humans. However, studies in rats at doses many times the recommended human dose have shown that use of enalapril causes the fetus to be smaller than normal. Studies in rabbits have shown that enalapril causes an increase in fetal death. Enalapril has not been shown to cause birth defects in rats or rabbits.

Studies with lisinopril have not been done in humans. However, studies in mice and rats at doses many times the recommended human dose have shown that use of lisinopril causes a decrease in successful pregnancies, a decrease in the weight of infants, and an increase in infant deaths. It has also caused a decrease in successful pregnancies and abnormal bone growth in rabbits. Lisinopril has not been shown to cause birth defects in mice, rats, or rabbits.

Be sure that you have discussed this with your doctor before taking this medicine.

—if you are **breast-feeding**. Captopril passes into the breast milk. It is not known whether enalapril or lisinopril passes into the breast milk. However, these medicines have not been shown to cause problems in nursing babies.

—if you have any of the following medical problems:

Diabetes mellitus (sugar diabetes)
Heart or blood vessel disease
Kidney disease
Liver disease
Systemic lupus erythematosus (SLE)

—if you have recently had a heart attack or stroke.

—if you have had a kidney transplant.

—if you are using **any** other prescription or nonprescription (OTC) medicine, especially one that contains:

Diuretics (water pills)
Potassium-containing medicines or supplements
Salt substitutes

Proper Use of This Medicine

To help you remember to take your medicine, try to get into the habit of taking it at the same time each day.

For patients taking captopril:

• This medicine is best taken on an empty stomach 1 hour before meals, unless you are otherwise directed by your doctor.

For patients taking this medicine for high blood pressure:

• Importance of diet—When prescribing medicine for your condition, your doctor may also prescribe a personal diet for you. Such a diet may be low in sodium (salt). Most people eat much more sodium than they need and too much sodium in the diet may increase blood pressure. Some foods that contain large amounts of sodium are canned soup, pickles, ketchup, green and ripe olives, relish, frankfurters, soy sauce, and carbonated beverages. Your doctor may want you to limit the amounts of these and other high-sodium foods in your diet. High blood pressure medicine is usually more effective when such a diet is properly followed.

However, too little sodium in the body can also cause problems when this medicine is taken. For example, blood pressure may be lowered more than is wanted. In addition, salt substitutes and low-salt milk may contain potassium, which may cause problems when taken with this medicine. Do not use these products unless told to do so by your doctor.

Also, it may be very important for you to go on a reducing diet. However, check with your doctor before changing your diet.

• Many patients who have high blood pressure will not notice any signs of the problem. In fact, many may feel normal. It is very important that you **take your medicine exactly as directed** and that you keep your appointments with your doctor even if you feel well.

• Remember that this medicine will not cure your high blood pressure but it does help control it. Therefore, you must continue to take it as directed if you expect to lower your blood pressure and keep it down. **You may have to take high blood pressure medicine for the rest of your life.** If high blood pressure is not treated, it can cause serious problems such as heart failure, blood vessel disease, stroke, or kidney disease.

If you miss a dose of this medicine, take it as soon as possible. However, if it is almost time for your next dose, skip the missed dose and go back to your regular dosing schedule. Do not double doses.

How to store this medicine:

• **Keep out of the reach of children.**

• Store away from heat and direct light.

• Do not store in the bathroom, near the kitchen sink, or in other damp places. Heat or moisture may cause the medicine to break down.

• Do not keep outdated medicine or medicine no longer needed. Be sure that any discarded medicine is out of the reach of children.

Precautions While Using This Medicine

It is important that your doctor check your progress at regular visits to make sure that this medicine is working properly and to check for unwanted effects.

For patients taking this medicine for high blood pressure:

  • **Do not take other medicines unless they have been discussed with your doctor.** This especially includes over-the-counter (nonprescription) medicines for appetite control, asthma, colds, cough, hay fever, or sinus problems, since they may tend to increase your blood pressure.

Dizziness or lightheadedness may occur after the first dose of this medicine, especially if you have been taking a diuretic (water pill). Make sure you know how you react to this medicine before you drive, use machines, or do other jobs that could be dangerous if you are not alert.

Check with your doctor right away if you become sick while taking this medicine, especially with severe or continuing nausea and vomiting or diarrhea. These conditions may cause you to lose too much water and lead to low blood pressure.

Dizziness, lightheadedness, or fainting may also occur if you exercise or if the weather is hot. Heavy sweating can cause loss of too much water and low blood pressure. Use extra care during exercise or hot weather.

Before having any kind of surgery (including dental surgery) or emergency treatment, tell the physician or dentist in charge that you are taking this medicine.

For patients taking captopril:

  • Tell the doctor in charge that you are taking this medicine before you have any medical tests. The results of some tests may be affected by this medicine.

Side Effects of This Medicine

Along with its needed effects, a medicine may cause some unwanted effects. Although not all of these side effects may occur, if they do occur they may need medical attention.

Check with your doctor immediately if any of the following side effects occur:

Rare

    Difficult breathing (sudden)
    Fever and chills
    Swelling of face, mouth, hands, or feet

Check with your doctor as soon as possible if any of the following side effects occur:

Less common

Dizziness, lightheadedness, or fainting
Skin rash, with or without itching, fever, or joint pain

Rare

Chest pain

Signs and symptoms of too much potassium in the body

Confusion
Irregular heartbeat
Numbness or tingling in hands, feet, or lips
Unexplained nervousness
Weakness or heaviness of legs

Other side effects may occur that usually do not require medical attention. These side effects may go away during treatment as your body adjusts to the medicine. However, check with your doctor if any of the following side effects continue or are bothersome:

Less common

Cough (dry, continuing)
Diarrhea
Headache
Loss of taste
Nausea
Unusual tiredness

For elderly patients:

• Some medicines may affect older patients differently than they do younger adults. Dizziness and lightheadedness may be more likely to occur in the elderly, who are sometimes more sensitive to the effects of this medicine. Check with your doctor if this continues or is bothersome. In addition, it is a good idea to check with your doctor or pharmacist if you notice any other unusual effects while taking this medicine or if you think it is not working as it should.

Other side effects not listed above may also occur in some patients. If you notice any other effects, check with your doctor.

ANGIOTENSIN-CONVERTING ENZYME (ACE) INHIBITORS AND HYDROCHLOROTHIAZIDE (Systemic)†

This information applies to the following medicines:

Captopril (KAP-toe-pril) and Hydrochlorothiazide (hye-droe-klor-oh-THYE-a-zide)

Enalapril (e-NAL-a-pril) and Hydrochlorothiazide

Some commonly used brand names in the U.S. are:

For Captopril and Hydrochlorothiazide†
Capozide

For Enalapril and Hydrochlorothiazide†
Vaseretic

†Not commercially available in Canada.

This combination belongs to the general class of medicines called antihypertensives. It is used to treat high blood pressure.

High blood pressure adds to the workload of the heart and arteries. If it continues for a long time, the heart and arteries may not function properly. This can damage the blood vessels of the brain, heart, and kidneys, resulting in a stroke, heart failure, or kidney failure. High blood pressure may also increase the risk of heart attacks. These problems may be less likely to occur if blood pressure is controlled.

The exact way in which captopril and enalapril work is not known. They block an enzyme in the body that is necessary to produce a substance that causes blood vessels to tighten. As a result, they probably relax blood vessels. This lowers blood pressure and increases the supply of blood and oxygen to the heart. Hydrochlorothiazide helps reduce the amount of salt and water in the body by acting on the kidneys to increase the flow of urine; this also helps to lower blood pressure.

This combination may also be used for other conditions as determined by your doctor.

This medicine is available only with doctor's prescription.

Before Using This Medicine

To decide on the best treatment for your medical problem, your doctor should be told:

—if you have ever had any unusual or allergic reaction to enalapril, captopril, sulfonamides (sulfa medicine), or hydrochlorothiazide or any of the other thiazide diuretics (water pills).

—if you are on a low-salt, low-sugar, or any other special diet, or if you are allergic to any substance, such as foods, sulfites or other preservatives, or dyes. Most medicines contain more than their active ingredient. Your doctor, nurse, or pharmacist can help you avoid products that may cause a problem.

—if you are **pregnant** or if you may become pregnant. Studies with this medicine have not been done in humans. In humans, captopril (contained in this combination medicine) has been reported to cause slowed growth of the fetus and difficult breathing and low blood pressure in the newborn. In addition, one case of a possible birth defect has been reported. Studies in rabbits and rats at doses up to 400 times the recommended human dose have shown that captopril causes an increase in death of the fetus and newborn. Also, captopril has caused deformed skulls in rabbits.

Studies in rats at doses many times the recommended human dose have shown that use of enalapril (contained in this combination medicine) causes the fetus to be smaller than normal. Studies in rabbits have shown that enalapril causes an increase in fetal death. This medicine has not been shown to cause birth defects in rats or rabbits.

Hydrochlorothiazide (contained in this combination medicine) has not been shown to cause birth defects or other problems in animal studies. However, when hydrochlorothiazide is used during pregnancy, it may cause side effects including jaundice, blood problems, and low potassium in the newborn baby.

Be sure that you have discussed this with your doctor before taking this medicine.

—if you are **breast-feeding**. Captopril and hydrochlorothiazide pass into breast milk. It is not known whether enalapril passes into breast milk. However, this medicine has not been shown to cause problems in nursing babies.

—if you have any of the following medical problems:

Diabetes mellitus (sugar diabetes)
Gout (or history of)
Heart or blood vessel disease
Kidney disease
Liver disease
Pancreatitis (inflammation of the pancreas)
Systemic lupus erythematosus (SLE) (or history of)

—if you have recently had a heart attack or stroke.

—if you have had a kidney transplant.

—if you are using **any** other prescription or nonprescription (OTC) medicine, especially one that contains:

Adrenocorticoids (cortisone-like medicine)
Digitalis glycosides (heart medicine)
Diuretics (water pills)Lithium (e.g., Lithane)
Methenamine (e.g., Mandelamine)
Potassium-containing medicines or supplements
Salt substitutes

Proper Use of This Medicine

To help you remember to take your medicine, try to get into the habit of taking it at the same time each day.

For patients taking captopril and hydrochlorothiazide:

• This medicine is best taken on an empty stomach 1 hour before meals, unless you are otherwise directed by your doctor.

For patients taking this medicine for high blood pressure:

• Importance of diet—When prescribing medicine for your condition, your doctor may also prescribe a personal diet for you. Such a diet may be low in sodium (salt). Most people eat much more sodium than they need and too much sodium in the diet may increase blood pressure. Some foods that contain large amounts of sodium are canned soup, pickles, ketchup, green and ripe olives, relish, frankfurters, soy sauce, and carbonated beverages. Your doctor may want you to limit the amounts of these and other high-sodium foods in your diet. High blood pressure medicine is usually more effective when such a diet is properly followed.

However, too little sodium in the body can also cause problems when this medicine is taken. For example, blood pressure may be lowered more than is wanted. In addition, salt substitutes and low-salt milk may contain potassium, which may cause problems when taken with this medicine. Do not use these products unless told to do so by your doctor.

Also, it may be very important for you to go on a reducing diet. However, check with your doctor before changing your diet.

• Many patients who have high blood pressure will not notice any signs of the problem. In fact, many may feel normal. It is very important that you **take your medicine exactly as directed** and that you keep your appointments with your doctor even if you feel well.

• Remember that this medicine will not cure your high blood pressure but it does help control it. Therefore, you must continue to take it as directed if you expect to lower your blood pressure and keep it down. **You may have to take high blood pressure medicine for the rest of your life.** If high blood pressure is not treated, it can cause serious problems such as heart failure, blood vessel disease, stroke, or kidney disease.

This medicine may cause you to have an unusual feeling or tiredness when you begin to take it. You may also notice an increase in the amount of urine or in your frequency of urination. After you have taken the medicine for a while, these effects should lessen. In general, to keep the increase in urine from affecting your nighttime sleep:

• If you are to take a single dose a day, take it in the morning after breakfast.

• If you are to take more than one dose a day, take the last dose no later than 6 p.m., unless otherwise directed by your doctor.

However, it is best to plan your dose or doses according to a schedule that will least affect your personal activities and sleep. Ask your doctor, nurse, or pharmacist to help you plan the best time to take this medicine.

If you miss a dose of this medicine, take it as soon as possible. However, if it is almost time for your next dose, skip the

missed dose and go back to your regular dosing schedule.
Do not double doses.

How to store this medicine:

- **Keep out of the reach of children.**

- Store away from heat and direct light.

- Do not store in the bathroom, near the kitchen sink, or in other damp places. Heat or moisture may cause the medicine to break down.

- Do not keep outdated medicine or medicine no longer needed. Be sure that any discarded medicine is out of the reach of children.

Precautions While Using This Medicine

It is important that your doctor check your progress at regular visits to make sure that this medicine is working properly and to check for unwanted effects.

Check with your doctor right away if you become sick while taking this medicine, especially with severe or continuing nausea and vomiting or diarrhea. These conditions may cause you to lose too much water and lead to low blood pressure.

Dizziness, lightheadedness, or fainting may also occur if you exercise or if the weather is hot. Heavy sweating can cause loss of too much water and low blood pressure. Use extra care during exercise or hot weather.

Before having any kind of surgery (including dental surgery) or emergency treatment, tell the physician or dentist in charge that you are taking this medicine.

For patients taking this medicine for high blood pressure:

- **Do not take other medicines unless they have been discussed with your doctor.** This especially includes over-the-counter (nonprescription) medicines for appetite control, asthma, colds, cough, hay fever, or sinus problems, since they may tend to increase your blood pressure.

For diabetic patients:

  • Hydrochlorothiazide (contained in this combination medicine) may raise blood sugar levels. While you are taking this medicine, be especially careful in testing for sugar in your urine.

Some people who take hydrochlorothiazide (contained in this combination medicine) may become more sensitive to sunlight than they are normally. When you first begin taking this medicine, avoid too much sun and do not use a sunlamp until you see how you react to the sun, especially if you tend to burn easily. If you have a severe reaction, check with your doctor.

Tell the doctor in charge that you are taking this medicine before you have any medical tests. The results of some tests may be affected by this medicine.

Side Effects of This Medicine

Along with its needed effects, a medicine may cause some unwanted effects. Although not all of these side effects may occur, if they do occur they may need medical attention.

Check with your doctor immediately if any of the following side effects occur:

Rare

  Difficult breathing (sudden)
  Fever and chills
  Swelling of face, mouth, hands, or feet

Check with your doctor as soon as possible if any of the following side effects occur:

Less common

  Dizziness, lightheadedness, or fainting
  Skin rash, with or without itching or fever

Rare

  Chest pain
  Joint, lower back or side, or stomach pain
  Stomach pain (severe) with nausea and vomiting
  Unusual bleeding or bruising
  Yellow eyes or skin

*Signs and symptoms of too much or too little potassium
in the body*

Dryness of mouth
Increased thirst
Irregular heartbeats
Mood or mental changes
Muscle cramps or pain
Numbness or tingling in hands, feet, or lips
Shortness of breath or difficult breathing
Weakness or heaviness of legs
Weak pulse

Other side effects may occur that usually do not require
medical attention. These side effects may go away
during treatment as your body adjusts to the medicine.
However, check with your doctor if any of the following side effects continue or are bothersome:

Less common

Cough (dry, continuing)
Diarrhea
Headache
Increased sensitivity of skin to sunlight
Loss of taste
Stomach upset
Unusual tiredness

For elderly patients:

• Some medicines may affect older patients differently than they do younger adults. Dizziness or lightheadedness and symptoms of too much potassium loss
may be more likely to occur in the elderly, who are
more sensitive to the effects of this medicine. Check
with your doctor if these continue or are bothersome.
In addition, it is a good idea to check with your doctor
or pharmacist if you notice any other unusual effects
or if you think it is not working as it should.

Other side effects not listed above may also occur in some
patients. If you notice any other effects, check with
your doctor.

BETA-ADRENERGIC BLOCKING AGENTS
(Systemic)

This information applies to the following medicines:

Acebutolol (a-se-BYOO-toe-lole)
Atenolol (a-TEN-oh-lole)
Carteolol (KAR-tee-oh-lole)
Labetalol (la-BET-a-lole)
Metoprolol (me-TOE-proe-lole)
Nadolol (NAY-doe-lole)
Oxprenolol (ox-PREN-oh-lole)
Penbutolol (pen-BYOO-toe-lole)
Pindolol (PIN-doe-lole)
Propranolol (proe-PRAN-oh-lole)
Sotalol (SOE-ta-lole)
Timolol (TIM-oh-lole)

Some commonly used brand names are:

For Acebutolol
In the U.S.
Sectral

In Canada
Monitan
Sectral

For Atenolol
In the U.S. and Canada
Tenormin

For Carteolol†
In the U.S.
Cartrol

For Labetalol
In the U.S.
Normodyne
Trandate

In Canada
Trandate

For Metoprolol
In the U.S.
Lopressor

In Canada
Apo-Metoprolol   Lopresor
Betaloc   Lopresor SR
Betaloc Durules   Novometoprol

Generic name product may also be available.

For Nadolol
In the U.S.
      Corgard
In Canada
      Corgard
  Generic name product may also be available.

For Oxprenolol*
In Canada
      Trasicor
      Slow-Trasicor

For Penbutolol†
In the U.S.
      Levatol

For Pindolol
In the U.S. and Canada
      Visken

For Propranolol
In the U.S.
      Inderal
      Inderal LA
  Generic name product may also be available.
In Canada

Apo-Propranolol	Inderal LA
Detensol	Novopranol
Inderal	pms Propranolol

  Generic name product may also be available.

For Sotalol*
In Canada
      Sotacor

For Timolol
In the U.S.
      Blocadren
In Canada
      Apo-Timol
      Blocadren

---

*Not commercially available in the U.S.

These medicines belong to a group of medicines known as beta-adrenergic blocking agents, beta-blocking agents, or more commonly, beta-blockers. Beta-blockers are used in the treatment of high blood pressure (hypertension). Some beta-blockers are also used to relieve angina (chest pain) and in heart attack patients to help prevent additional heart attacks. Beta-blockers have also been found useful in a number of other conditions such as correcting irregular heartbeats and preventing migraine headaches. They may also be used for other conditions as determined by your doctor.

Beta-blockers work by affecting the response to some nerve impulses in certain parts of the body. As a result, they decrease the need for blood and oxygen by the heart by reducing its workload. They also help the heart to beat more regularly.

Beta-adrenergic blocking agents are available only with your doctor's prescription.

Before Using This Medicine

To decide on the best treatment for your medical problem, your doctor should be told:

—if you have ever had any unusual or allergic reaction to beta-blocker medicine.

—if you are on a low-salt, low-sugar, or any other special diet, or if you are allergic to any substance, such as foods, sulfites or other preservatives, or dyes. Most medicines contain more than their active ingredient. Your doctor, nurse, or pharmacist can help you avoid products that may cause a problem.

—if you are **pregnant** or if you may become pregnant. Adequate studies have not been done in humans. However, use of some beta-blockers during pregnancy has been associated with breathing problems and a lower heart rate in the newborn infant. Some reports have shown no unwanted effects on the newborn infant. Animal studies have shown some beta-blockers to cause problems in pregnancy when used in doses many times the usual human dose.

—if you are **breast-feeding**. Although beta-blockers pass into the breast milk, these medicines have not been shown to cause problems in nursing babies.

—if you have any of the following medical problems:
    Allergy, history of (asthma, eczema, hay fever, hives)
    Bradycardia (unusually slow heartbeat)
    Bronchitis
    Diabetes mellitus (sugar diabetes)
    Emphysema

Heart or blood vessel disease
Kidney disease
Liver disease
Mental depression (or history of)
Myasthenia gravis (a muscle disease)
Overactive thyroid
Pheochromocytoma
Psoriasis

—if you are now taking or have taken within the past 2 weeks monoamine oxidase (MAO) inhibitors such as:

Furazolidone (e.g., Furoxone)
Isocarboxazid (e.g., Marplan)
Pargyline (e.g., Eutonyl)
Phenelzine (e.g., Nardil)
Procarbazine (e.g., Matulane)
Tranylcypromine (e.g., Parnate)

—if you are taking **any** other prescription or nonprescription (OTC) medicine, especially one that contains:

Aminophylline (e.g., Somophyllin)
Antidiabetics, oral (diabetes medicine you take by mouth)
Caffeine (e.g., NoDoz)
Clonidine (e.g., Catapres)
Diltiazem (e.g., Cardizem)
Dyphylline (e.g., Lufyllin)
Guanabenz (e.g., Wytensin)
Insulin
Nifedipine (e.g., Procardia)
Oxtriphylline (e.g., Choledyl)
Theophylline (e.g., Somophyllin-T)
Verapamil (e.g., Calan)

—if you smoke.

Proper Use of This Medicine

For patients taking the extended-release capsule or tablet form of this medicine:

• Swallow the capsule or tablet whole.

• Do not crush, break, or chew before swallowing.

Ask your doctor about checking your pulse rate before and after taking beta-blocking agents. Then, while you are taking this medicine, check your pulse regularly. If it is much slower than your usual rate (or less than 50 beats per minute), check with your doctor. A pulse rate that is too slow may cause circulation problems.

To help you remember to take your medicine, try to get into the habit of taking it at the same time each day.

For patients taking this medicine for high blood pressure:

• Importance of diet—When prescribing medicine for your condition, your doctor may also prescribe a personal diet for you. Such a diet may be low in sodium (salt). Most people eat much more sodium than they need. Too much sodium in the diet may increase blood pressure. Some foods that contain large amounts of sodium are canned soup, pickles, ketchup, green and ripe olives, relish, frankfurters, soy sauce, and carbonated beverages. Your doctor may want you to limit the amounts of these and other high-sodium foods in your diet. High blood pressure medicine is usually more effective when such a diet is properly followed.

Also, it may be very important for you to go on a reducing diet. However, check with your doctor before changing your diet.

• Many patients who have high blood pressure will not notice any signs of the problem. In fact, many may feel normal. It is very important that you **take your medicine exactly as directed**. Also, keep your appointments with your doctor even if you feel well.

• Remember that this medicine will not cure your high blood pressure but it does help control it. Therefore, you must continue to take it as directed if you expect to lower your blood pressure and keep it down. **You may have to take high blood pressure medicine for the rest of your life.** If high blood pressure is not treated, it can cause serious problems such as heart failure, blood vessel disease, stroke, or kidney disease.

Do not miss any doses. This is especially important when you are taking only one dose per day. Some conditions may become worse when this medicine is not taken regularly.

If you do miss a dose of this medicine, take it as soon as possible. However, if it is within 4 hours of your next dose (8 hours when using atenolol, carteolol, labetalol, nadolol, penbutolol, sotalol, or extended-release oxprenolol or propranolol), skip the missed dose and go back to your regular dosing schedule. Do not double doses.

How to store this medicine:

• **Keep out of the reach of children.**

• Store away from heat and direct light.

• Do not store in the bathroom, near the kitchen sink, or in other damp places. Heat or moisture may cause the medicine to break down.

• Do not keep outdated medicine or medicine no longer needed. Be sure that any discarded medicine is out of the reach of children.

Precautions While Using This Medicine

It is important that your doctor check your progress at regular visits. This is to make sure the medicine is working for you and to allow the dosage to be changed if needed.

Do not stop taking this medicine without first checking with your doctor. Your doctor may want you to reduce gradually the amount you are taking before stopping completely. Some conditions may become worse when the medicine is stopped suddenly, and danger of heart attack is increased in some patients.

Make sure that you have enough medicine on hand to last through weekends, holidays, or vacations. You may want to carry an extra written prescription in your billfold or purse in case of an emergency. You can then have it filled if you run out of medicine while you are away from home.

Your doctor may want you to carry a medical identification card stating that you are taking this medicine.

Before having any kind of surgery (including dental surgery) or emergency treatment, tell the physician or dentist in charge that you are taking this medicine.

For diabetic patients:

• **This medicine may cause your blood sugar levels to fall.** Also, **this medicine may cover up signs of hypoglycemia (low blood sugar),** such as change in pulse rate.

This medicine may cause some people to become dizzy, drowsy, lightheaded, or less alert than they are normally. **Make sure you know how you react to this medicine before you drive, use machines, or do other jobs that could be dangerous if you are not alert.** If the problem continues or gets worse, check with your doctor.

Beta-blockers may make you more sensitive to cold temperatures. They tend to decrease blood circulation in the skin, fingers, and toes. Dress warmly during cold weather and be careful during prolonged exposure to cold, such as in winter sports.

Chest pain resulting from exercise or physical exertion is usually reduced or prevented by this medicine. This may tempt a patient to be overly active. **Make sure you discuss with your doctor a safe amount of exercise for your medical problem.**

Tell the doctor in charge that you are taking this medicine before you have any medical tests. The results of some tests may be affected by this medicine.

For patients with allergies to foods, medicines, or insect stings:
• There is a chance that this medicine will cause allergic reactions to be worse and harder to treat. If you have a severe allergic reaction while you are being treated with this medicine, check with a doctor right away so that it can be treated.

For patients taking this medicine for high blood pressure:
• **Do not take other medicines unless they have been discussed with your doctor.** This especially includes over-the-counter (nonprescription) medicines for appetite control, asthma, colds, cough, hay fever, or sinus problems since they may tend to increase your blood pressure.

For patients taking labetalol by mouth:
• **Dizziness, lightheadedness, or fainting may occur, especially when you get up from a lying or sitting position.** This is more likely to occur when you first start taking labetalol or when the dose is increased. **Getting up slowly may help.** When you get up from lying down, sit on the

edge of the bed with your feet dangling for 1 to 2 minutes. Then stand up slowly. If the problem continues or gets worse, check with your doctor.

• The dizziness, lightheadedness, or fainting is also more likely to occur if you drink alcohol, stand for long periods of time, exercise, or if the weather is hot. **While you are taking this medicine, be careful in the amount of alcohol you drink. Also, use extra care during exercise or hot weather or if you must stand for long periods of time.**

For patients receiving labetalol by injection:

• It is very important that you lie down flat while receiving labetalol and for up to 3 hours afterward. If you try to get up too soon, you may become dizzy or faint. **Do not try to sit or stand until your doctor tells you to do so.**

Side Effects of This Medicine

Along with its needed effects, a medicine may cause some unwanted effects. Although not all of these side effects may occur, if they do occur they may need medical attention.

Check with your doctor as soon as possible if any of the following side effects occur:

Less common

Breathing difficulty and/or wheezing
Cold hands and feet
Confusion (especially in elderly)
Hallucinations (seeing, hearing, or feeling things that are not there)
Irregular heartbeat
Mental depression
Nightmares and vivid dreams
Skin rash
Slow heartbeat (especially less than 50 beats per minute)— more common with nadolol, propranolol, and sotalol; rare with labetalol, penbutolol, and pindolol
Swelling of ankles, feet, and/or lower legs

Rare

Back pain or joint pain—more common with pindolol
Chest pain

Fever and sore throat
Red, scaling, or crusted skin
Unusual bleeding and bruising

Signs and symptoms of overdose (in the order in which they may occur)

Slow heartbeat
Dizziness (severe) or fainting
Fast or irregular heartbeat
Difficulty in breathing
Bluish-colored fingernails or palms of hands
Convulsions (seizures)

Other side effects may occur that usually do not require medical attention. These side effects may go away during treatment as your body adjusts to the medicine. However, check with your doctor if any of the following side effects continue or are bothersome:

More common

Decreased sexual ability
Dizziness or lightheadedness
Drowsiness (slight)
Trouble in sleeping
Unusual tiredness or weakness

Less common or rare

Anxiety and/or nervousness
Changes in taste—for labetalol only
Constipation
Diarrhea
Dry, sore eyes
Frequent urination—for acebutolol only
Itching of skin
Nausea or vomiting
Numbness and/or tingling of fingers and/or toes
Numbness and/or tingling of skin, especially on scalp—for labetalol only
Stomach discomfort
Stuffy nose

Although not all of the side effects listed above have been reported for all of these medicines, they have been reported for at least one of them. Since all of the beta-adrenergic blocking agents are very similar, any of the above side effects may occur with any of these medicines. However, they may be more or less common with some agents than with others.

After you have been taking a beta-blocker for a while, it may cause unpleasant or even harmful effects if you stop taking it too suddenly. After you stop taking this medicine or while you are gradually reducing the amount you are taking, check with your doctor right away if any of the following occur:

> Chest pain
> Fast or irregular heartbeat
> General feeling of body discomfort or weakness
> Shortness of breath (sudden)
> Sweating
> Trembling

For elderly patients:

- Some medicines may affect older patients differently than they do younger adults. Some of the above side effects are more likely to occur in the elderly, who are usually more sensitive to the effects of beta-blockers. Check with your doctor if these continue or are bothersome. In addition, it is a good idea to check with your doctor or pharmacist if you notice any other unusual effects while taking this medicine or if you think it is not working as it should.

For patients taking labetalol:

- You may notice a tingling feeling on your scalp when you first begin to take labetalol. This is to be expected and usually goes away after you have been taking labetalol for a while.

Other side effects not listed above may also occur in some patients. If you notice any other effects, check with your doctor.

BETA-ADRENERGIC BLOCKING AGENTS AND THIAZIDE DIURETICS
(Systemic)

This information applies to the following medicines:

Atenolol (a-TEN-oh-lole) and Chlorthalidone (klor-THAL-i-doan)
Labetalol (la-BET-a-lole) and Hydrochlorothiazide (hye-droe-klor-oh-THYE-a-zide)
Metoprolol (me-TOE-proe-lole) and Hydrochlorothiazide
Nadolol (NAY-doe-lole) and Bendroflumethiazide (ben-droe-floo-meth-EYE-a-zide)
Pindolol (PIN-doe-lole) and Hydrochlorothiazide
Propranolol (proe-PRAN-oh-lole) and Hydrochlorothiazide
Timolol (TIM-oh-lole) and Hydrochlorothiazide

Some commonly used brand names are:

For Atenolol and Chlorthalidone†
In the U.S.
　　Tenoretic

For Labetalol and Hydrochlorothiazide†
In the U.S.
　　Normozide
　　Trandate HCT

For Metoprolol and Hydrochlorothiazide
In the U.S.
　　Lopressor HCT

In Canada
　　Co-Betaloc

For Nadolol and Bendroflumethiazide
In the U.S. and Canada
　　Corzide

For Pindolol and Hydrochlorothiazide*
In Canada
　　Viskazide

For Propranolol and Hydrochlorothiazide
In the U.S.
　　Inderide
　　Inderide LA

　　Generic name product may also be available.

In Canada
　　Inderide

For Timolol and Hydrochlorothiazide
In the U.S. and Canada
Timolide

---

*Not commercially available in the U.S.
†Not commercially available in Canada.

Beta-blocker and thiazide diuretic combinations belong to the group of medicines known as antihypertensives (blood pressure medicine). Both ingredients of the combination control high blood pressure, but work in different ways. Beta-blockers (atenolol, labetalol, metoprolol, nadolol, pindolol, propranolol, and timolol) reduce the workload on the heart as well as having other effects. Thiazide diuretics (bendroflumethiazide, chlorthalidone, and hydrochlorothiazide) reduce the amount of fluid pressure in the body by increasing the flow of urine.

High blood pressure adds to the workload of the heart and arteries. If it continues for a long time, the heart and arteries may not function properly. This can damage the blood vessels of the brain, heart, and kidneys, resulting in a stroke, heart failure, or kidney failure. High blood pressure may also increase the risk of heart attacks. These problems may be less likely to occur if blood pressure is controlled.

Beta-blocker and thiazide diuretic combinations are available only with your doctor's prescription.

Before Using This Medicine

To decide on the best treatment for your medical problem, your doctor should be told:

—if you have ever had any unusual or allergic reaction to beta-blockers, sulfonamides (sulfa drugs), bumetanide, furosemide, acetazolamide, dichlorphenamide, methazolamide or to any of the thiazide diuretics.

—if you are on a low-salt, low-sugar, or any other special diet, or if you are allergic to any substance, such as foods, sulfites or other preservatives, or dyes. Most medicines contain more than their active ingredient. Your doctor, nurse, or pharmacist can help you avoid products that may cause a problem.

—if you are **pregnant** or if you may become pregnant. Although adequate studies in humans have not been done, use of some beta-blockers during pregnancy has been associated with breathing problems and a slower heart rate in the newborn infant. However, other reports have shown no unwanted effects in the newborn infant. Animal studies have shown some beta-blockers to cause problems in pregnancy when used in doses many times the usual human dose.

Studies with thiazide diuretics have not been done in humans. However, use during pregnancy may cause side effects such as jaundice, blood problems, and low potassium in the newborn infant. Animal studies have not shown thiazide diuretic medicines to cause birth defects even when used in doses several times the usual human dose.

—if you are **breast-feeding**. Although beta-blockers and thiazide diuretics pass into the breast milk, these medicines have not been shown to cause problems in nursing babies.

—if you have any of the following medical problems:

   Allergy, history of (asthma, eczema, hay fever, hives)
   Bradycardia (unusually slow heartbeat)
   Bronchitis
   Diabetes mellitus (sugar diabetes)
   Emphysema
   Gout (history of)
   Heart or blood vessel disease
   Kidney disease
   Liver disease
   Lupus erythematosus (history of)
   Mental depression (or history of)
   Myasthenia gravis (a muscle disease)
   Overactive thyroid
   Pancreatitis (inflammation of the pancreas)
   Pheochromocytoma
   Psoriasis

—if you are now taking or have taken within the past 2 weeks monoamine oxidase (MAO) inhibitors such as:

   Furazolidone (e.g., Furoxone)
   Isocarboxazid (e.g., Marplan)
   Pargyline (e.g., Eutonyl)
   Phenelzine (e.g., Nardil)
   Procarbazine (e.g., Matulane)
   Tranylcypromine (e.g., Parnate)

—if you are taking **any** other prescription or nonprescription (OTC) medicine, especially one that contains:

Adrenocorticoids (cortisone-like medicines)
Aminophylline (e.g., Somophyllin)
Antidiabetics, oral (diabetes medicine you take by mouth)
Caffeine (e.g., NoDoz)
Clonidine (e.g., Catapres)
Digitalis glycosides (heart medicine)
Diltiazem (e.g., Cardizem)
Dyphylline (e.g., Lufylline)
Guanabenz (e.g., Wytensin)
Insulin
Lithium (e.g., Lithane)
Methenamine (e.g., Mandelamine)
Nifedipine (e.g., Procardia)
Oxtriphylline (e.g., Choledyl)
Theophylline (e.g., Somophyllin-T)
Verapamil (e.g., Calan)

—if you smoke.

Proper Use of This Medicine

Importance of diet—When prescribing medicine for your condition, your doctor may also prescribe a personal diet for you. Such a diet may be low in sodium (salt). Most people eat much more sodium than they need. Too much sodium in the diet may increase blood pressure. Some foods that contain large amounts of sodium are canned soup, pickles, ketchup, green and ripe olives, relish, frankfurters, soy sauce, and carbonated beverages. Your doctor may want you to limit the amounts of these and other high-sodium foods in your diet. High blood pressure medicine is usually more effective when such a diet is properly followed.

Also, it may be very important for you to go on a reducing diet. However, check with your doctor before changing your diet.

Many patients who have high blood pressure will not notice any signs of the problem. In fact, many may feel normal. It is very important that you **take your medicine exactly as directed**. Also, keep your appointments with your doctor even if you feel well.

Remember that this medicine will not cure your high blood pressure but it does help control it. Therefore, you must continue to take it as directed if you expect to lower your blood pressure and keep it down. **You may have to take high blood pressure medicine for the rest of your life.** If high blood pressure is not treated, it can cause serious problems such as heart failure, blood vessel disease, stroke, or kidney disease.

For patients taking the extended-release tablet form of this medicine:

• Swallow the tablet whole.

• Do not crush, break, or chew before swallowing.

To help you remember to take your medicine, try to get into the habit of taking it at the same time each day.

Ask your doctor about checking your pulse rate before and after taking beta-blocking agents. Then, while you are taking this medicine, check your pulse regularly. If it is much slower than your usual rate (or less than 50 beats per minute), check with your doctor. A pulse rate that is too slow may cause circulation problems.

The thiazide diuretic (e.g., bendroflumethiazide, chlorthalidone, or hydrochlorothiazide) contained in this combination medicine may cause you to have an unusual feeling of tiredness when you begin to take it. You may also notice an increase in the amount of urine or in your frequency of urination. After you take the medicine for a while, these effects should lessen. To keep the increase in urine from affecting your nighttime sleep:

• If you are to take a single dose a day, take it in the morning after breakfast.

• If you are to take more than one dose a day, take the last dose no later than 6 p.m., unless otherwise directed by your doctor.

However, it is best to plan your dose or doses according to a schedule that will least affect your personal activities and sleep. Ask your doctor, nurse, or pharmacist to help you plan the best time to take this medicine.

Do not miss any doses. This is especially important when you are taking only one dose per day. Some conditions may become worse when this medicine is not taken regularly.

If you do miss a dose of this medicine, take it as soon as possible. However, if it is within 4 hours of your next dose (8 hours when using atenolol and chlorthalidone, labetalol and hydrochlorothiazide, nadolol and bendroflumethiazide, or extended-release propranolol and hydrochlorothiazide), skip the missed dose and go back to your regular dosing schedule. Do not double doses.

How to store this medicine:

- **Keep out of the reach of children.**

- Store away from heat and direct light.

- Do not store in the bathroom, near the kitchen sink, or in other damp places. Heat or moisture may cause the medicine to break down.

- Do not keep outdated medicine or medicine no longer needed. Be sure that any discarded medicine is out of the reach of children.

Precautions While Using This Medicine

It is important that your doctor check your progress at regular visits. This is to make sure the medicine is properly controlling your blood pressure and to allow the dosage to be changed if needed.

Do not stop taking this medicine without first checking with your doctor. Your doctor may want you to reduce gradually the amount you are taking before stopping completely. Some conditions may become worse when the medicine is stopped suddenly, and the risk of heart attack is increased in some patients.

Make sure that you have enough medicine on hand to last through weekends, holidays, or vacations. You may want to carry an extra written prescription in your billfold or purse in case of an emergency. You can then have it filled if you run out of medicine while you are away from home.

Your doctor may want you to carry a medical identification card stating that you are taking this medicine.

**Do not take other medicines unless they have been discussed
with your doctor.** This especially includes over-the-counter
(nonprescription) medicines for appetite control, asthma,
colds, cough, hay fever, or sinus problems since they may
tend to increase your blood pressure.

**Before having any kind of surgery (including dental surgery)
or emergency treatment, tell the physician or dentist in
charge that you are taking this medicine.**

For diabetic patients:

 • **This medicine may cause your blood sugar levels to rise
or to fall.** Also, **this medicine may cover up signs of hypoglycemia (low blood sugar),** such as change in pulse rate.
While you are taking this medicine, be especially careful
in testing for sugar in your urine. If you have any questions about this, check with your doctor.

**The thiazide diuretic contained in this medicine may cause
a loss of potassium from your body.**
 • To help prevent this, your doctor may want you to:
 —eat or drink foods that have a high potassium content (for example, orange or other citrus fruit juices),
or

 —take a potassium supplement, or

 —take another medicine to help prevent the loss of
the potassium in the first place.

 • It is very important to follow these directions. Also, it
is important not to change your diet on your own. This
is more important if you are already on a special diet (as
for diabetes), or if you are taking a potassium supplement
or a medicine to reduce potassium loss. Extra potassium
may not be necessary and, in some cases, too much potassium could be harmful.

Check with your doctor if you become sick and have severe
or continuing vomiting or diarrhea. These problems may
cause you to lose additional water and potassium.

This medicine may cause some people to become dizzy,
drowsy, lightheaded, or less alert than they are normally.
Make sure you know how you react to this medicine before

you drive, use machines, or do other jobs that could be dangerous if you are not alert. If the problem continues or gets worse, check with your doctor.

The beta-blocker (atenolol, labetalol, metoprolol, nadolol, pindolol, propranolol, or timolol) contained in this medicine may make you more sensitive to cold temperatures. It tends to decrease blood circulation in the skin, fingers, and toes. Dress warmly during cold weather and be careful during prolonged exposure to cold, such as in winter sports.

Some people who take this medicine may become more sensitive to sunlight than they are normally. When you begin taking this medicine, avoid too much sun and do not use a sunlamp until you see how you react to the sun, especially if you tend to burn easily. If you have a severe reaction, check with your doctor.

Tell the doctor in charge that you are taking this medicine before you have any medical tests. The results of some tests may be affected by this medicine.

For patients with allergies to foods, medicines, or insect stings:
 • There is a chance that this medicine will cause allergic reactions to be worse and harder to treat. If you have a severe allergic reaction while you are being treated with this medicine, check with a doctor right away so that it can be treated.

Side Effects of This Medicine

Along with its needed effects, a medicine may cause some unwanted effects. Although not all of these side effects may occur, if they do occur they may need medical attention.

Check with your doctor as soon as possible if any of the following side effects occur:
Less common
    Breathing difficulty and/or wheezing
    Cold hands and feet
    Confusion (especially in elderly)

Hallucinations (seeing, hearing, or feeling things that are not there)
Irregular heartbeat
Mental depression
Slow pulse (especially less than 50 beats per minute)

Rare

Chest pain
Fever and sore throat
Joint, side, or stomach pain
Red, scaling, or crusted skin
Skin rash or hives
Stomach pain (severe) with nausea and vomiting
Unusual bleeding or bruising
Yellow eyes or skin

Signs of too much potassium loss

Dryness of mouth
Increased thirst
Irregular heartbeats
Mood or mental changes
Muscle cramps or pain
Weak pulse

Signs and symptoms of overdose (in the order in which they may occur)

Slow heartbeat
Dizziness (severe) or fainting
Difficulty in breathing
Bluish-colored fingernails or palms of hands
Convulsions (seizures)

Other side effects may occur that usually do not require medical attention. These side effects may go away during treatment as your body adjusts to the medicine. However, check with your doctor if any of the following side effects continue or are bothersome:

More common

Decreased sexual ability
Dizziness or lightheadedness
Drowsiness (slight)
Trouble in sleeping
Unusual tiredness or weakness

Less common

Anxiety or nervousness
Changes in taste—for labctalol and hydrochlorothiazide only

Constipation
Diarrhea
Dry, sore eyes
Increased sensitivity of skin to sunlight
Itching of skin
Loss of appetite
Nausea or vomiting
Nightmares and vivid dreams
Numbness and/or tingling of skin, especially on scalp—for
    labetalol and hydrochlorothiazide only
Numbness or tingling of fingers and toes
Stomach discomfort or upset
Stuffy nose

Although not all of the above side effects have been reported for all of these medicines, they have been reported for at least one of the beta-adrenergic blockers
or thiazide diuretics. Since all of the beta-adrenergic
blocking agents are very similar and the thiazide diuretics are also very similar, any of the above side
effects may occur with any of these medicines. However, they may be more common with some combinations than with others.

After you have been taking this medicine for a while, it
may cause unpleasant or even harmful effects if you
stop taking it too suddenly. After you stop taking this
medicine or while you are gradually reducing the
amount you are taking, check with your doctor right
away if any of the following occur:

Chest pain
Fast or irregular heartbeat
General feeling of body discomfort or weakness
Headache
Shortness of breath (sudden)
Sweating
Trembling

For elderly patients:

• Some medicines may affect older patients differently
than they do younger adults. Some of the above side
effects, especially dizziness or lightheadedness and signs
of too much potassium loss, may be more likely to occur

in the elderly, who are usually more sensitive to the effects of this medicine. Check with your doctor if these occur. In addition, it is a good idea to check with your doctor or pharmacist if you notice any other unusual effects or if you think it is not working as it should.

Other side effects not listed above may also occur in some patients. If you notice any other effects, check with your doctor.

CALCIUM CHANNEL BLOCKING AGENTS
(Systemic)

This information applies to the following medicines:

Diltiazem (dil-TYE-a-zem)
Nifedipine (nye-FED-i-peen)
Verapamil (ver-AP-a-mil)

Some commonly used brand names are:

For Diltiazem
In the U.S.
Cardizem

In Canada
Cardizem

Generic name product may also be available.

For Nifedipine
In the U.S.
Adalat
Procardia

In Canada
Adalat   Apo-Nifed
Adalat P.A.   Novo-Nifedin

For Verapamil
In the U.S.
Calan   Isoptin
Calan SR   Isoptin SR

Generic name product may also be available.

In Canada
Isoptin

Diltiazem, nifedipine, and verapamil belong to the group of medicines called calcium channel blockers. They are taken by mouth or given by injection to relieve and control angina (chest pain).

Calcium channel blocking agents affect the movement of calcium into the cells of the heart and blood vessels. As a result, they relax blood vessels and increase the supply of blood and oxygen to the heart while reducing its work load.

Some of these medicines are also used to treat high blood pressure. High blood pressure adds to the workload of the heart and arteries. If it continues for a long time, the heart and arteries may not function properly. This can damage the blood vessels of the brain, heart, and kidneys, resulting in a stroke, heart failure, or kidney failure. High blood pressure may also increase the risk of heart attacks. These problems may be less likely to occur if blood pressure is controlled.

Calcium channel blocking agents may also be used for other conditions as determined by your doctor.

These medicines are available only with your doctor's prescription.

Before Using This Medicine

To decide on the best treatment for your medical problem, your doctor should be told:

—if you have ever had any unusual or allergic reaction to diltiazem, nifedipine, or verapamil.

—if you are on a low-salt, low-sugar, or any other special diet, or if you are allergic to any substance, such as foods, sulfites or other preservatives, or dyes. Most medicines contain more than their active ingredient. Your doctor, nurse, or pharmacist can help you avoid products that may cause a problem.

—if you are **pregnant** or if you may become pregnant. Studies have not been done in humans. However, studies in animals have shown that large doses of calcium channel blockers cause birth defects, prolonged pregnancy, poor bone development, and stillbirth.

—if you are **breast-feeding**. Although these medicines may pass into breast milk, they have not been shown to cause problems in nursing babies.

—if you have any of the following medical problems:
    Kidney disease
    Liver disease
    Other heart or blood vessel disorders

—if you are taking **any** other prescription or nonprescription (OTC) medicine, especially one that contains:
    Beta-blockers (acebutolol [e.g., Sectral], atenolol [e.g., Tenormin], labetalol [e.g., Normodyne], metoprolol [e.g., Lopressor], nadolol [e.g., Corgard], oxprenolol [e.g., Trasicor], pindolol [e.g., Visken], propranolol [e.g., Inderal], sotalol [e.g., Sotacor], timolol [e.g., Blocadren])
    Carbamazepine (e.g., Tegretol)
    Cyclosporine (e.g., Sandimmune)
    Digitalis glycosides (heart medicine)
    Disopyramide (e.g., Norpace)
    Quinidine (e.g., Quinidex)

Proper Use of This Medicine

Take this medicine exactly as directed even if you feel well and do not notice any signs of chest pain. Do not take more of this medicine and do not take it more often than your doctor ordered. Do not miss any doses.

For patients taking extended-release verapamil tablets:

• Swallow the tablet whole, without crushing or chewing it. However, if your doctor tells you to, you may break the tablet in half.

• Take the medicine with food or milk.

For patients taking this medicine for high blood pressure:

• Importance of diet—When prescribing medicine for your condition, your doctor may also prescribe a personal diet for you. Such a diet may be low in sodium (salt). Most people eat much more sodium than they need and too much sodium in the diet may increase blood pressure. Some foods that contain large amounts of sodium are canned soup, pickles, ketchup, green and ripe olives, relish, frankfurters, soy sauce, and carbonated beverages. Your doctor may want you to limit the amounts of these and other high-sodium foods in your diet. High blood pressure medicine is usually more effective when such a diet is properly followed.

Also, it may be very important for you to go on a reducing diet. However, check with your doctor before changing your diet.

• Many patients who have high blood pressure will not notice any signs of the problem. In fact, many may feel normal. It is very important that you **take your medicine exactly as directed** and that you keep your appointments with your doctor even if you feel well.

• Remember that this medicine will not cure your high blood pressure but it does help control it. Therefore, you must continue to take it as directed if you expect to lower your blood pressure and keep it down. **You may have to take high blood pressure medicine for the rest of your life.** If high blood pressure is not treated, it can cause serious problems such as heart failure, blood vessel disease, stroke, or kidney disease.

If you do miss a dose of this medicine, take it as soon as possible. However, if it is almost time for your next dose, skip the missed dose and go back to your regular dosing schedule. Do not double doses.

How to store this medicine:

• **Keep out of the reach of children.**

• Store away from heat and direct light.

• Do not store in the bathroom, near the kitchen sink, or in other damp places. Heat or moisture may cause the medicine to break down.

• Do not keep outdated medicine or medicine no longer needed. Be sure that any discarded medicine is out of the reach of children.

Precautions While Using This Medicine

It is important that your doctor check your progress at regular visits. This will allow your doctor to make sure the medicine is working properly and to change the dosage if needed.

If you have been using this medicine regularly for several weeks, do not suddenly stop using it. Stopping suddenly may bring on attacks of angina. Check with your doctor for the best way to reduce gradually the amount you are taking before stopping completely.

Dizziness, lightheadedness, or a fainting feeling may occur, especially when you get up quickly from a lying or sitting position. Getting up slowly may help. **Also, drinking alcohol may make these effects worse and may cause a serious drop in blood pressure.** Check with your doctor before drinking alcoholic beverages while you are taking this medicine.

Chest pain resulting from exercise or physical exertion is usually reduced or prevented by this medicine. This may tempt you to be overly active. **Make sure you discuss with your doctor a safe amount of exercise for your medical problem.**

After taking a dose of this medicine you may get a headache that lasts for a short time. This effect is more common if you are taking nifedipine. This should become less noticeable after you have taken this medicine for a while. If this effect continues or if the headaches are severe, check with your doctor.

In some patients, tenderness, swelling, or bleeding of the gums may appear soon after this treatment with this medicine is started. Brushing and flossing your teeth carefully and regularly and massaging your gums may help prevent this. **See your dentist regularly to have your teeth cleaned. Check with your physician or dentist if you have any questions about how to take care of your teeth and gums, or if you notice any tenderness, swelling, or bleeding of your gums.**

For patients taking diltiazem or verapamil:

• **Ask your doctor how to count your pulse rate. Then, while you are taking this medicine, check your pulse regularly.** If it is much slower than your usual rate, or less than 50 beats per minute, check with your doctor. A pulse rate that is too slow may cause circulation problems.

For patients taking this medicine for high blood pressure:

• **Do not take other medicines unless they have been discussed with your doctor.** This especially includes over-the-counter (nonprescription) medicines for appetite control, asthma, colds, cough, hay fever, or sinus problems, since they may tend to increase your blood pressure.

Side Effects of This Medicine

Along with its needed effects, a medicine may cause some unwanted effects. Although not all of these side effects may occur, if they do occur they may need medical attention.

Check with your doctor as soon as possible if any of the following side effects occur:

Less common

   Breathing difficulty, coughing, or wheezing
   Irregular or fast, pounding heartbeat

Skin rash
Slow heartbeat (less than 50 beats per minute—diltiazem
and verapamil only)
Swelling of ankles, feet, or lower legs (more common with
nifedipine)

Rare

Bleeding, tender, or swollen gums
Chest pain (may appear about 30 minutes after nifedipine
is taken)
Fainting

Other side effects may occur that usually do not require
medical attention. These side effects may go away
during treatment as your body adjusts to the medicine.
However, check with your doctor if any of the following side effects continue or are bothersome:

Less common or rare

Constipation
Dizziness or lightheadedness (more common with nifedipine)
Flushing and feeling of warmth (more common with nifed-
ipine)
Headache (more common with nifedipine)
Nausea (more common with nifedipine)
Nervousness or mood changes
Shakiness or weakness
Stomach cramps
Stuffy nose
Unusual tiredness

Although not all of the side effects listed above have been
reported for all of these medicines, they have been
reported for at least one of them. Since some of the
effects of calcium channel blockers are similar, some
of the above side effects may occur with any of these
medicines. However, they may be more common with
some of these medicines than with others.

For elderly patients:

• Some medicines may affect older patients differently than they do younger adults. The above side
effects may be more likely to occur in the elderly, who
are usually more sensitive to this medicine. Check with

your doctor if this occurs. In addition, it is a good idea to check with your doctor or pharmacist if you notice any other unusual effects while taking this medicine or if you think it is not working as it should.

Other side effects not listed above may also occur in some patients. If you notice any other effects, check with your doctor.

CLONIDINE (Systemic)

Some commonly used brand names are:

In the U.S.

      Catapres

      Catapres-TTS

    Generic name product may also be available.

In Canada

      Catapres

      Dixarit

Clonidine (KLOE-ni-deen) belongs to the general class of medicines called antihypertensives. It is used to treat high blood pressure.

High blood pressure adds to the workload of the heart and arteries. If it continues for a long time, the heart and arteries may not function properly. This can damage the blood vessels of the brain, heart, and kidneys, resulting in a stroke, heart failure, or kidney failure. Hypertension may also increase the risk of heart attacks. These problems may be less likely to occur if blood pressure is controlled.

Clonidine works by controlling nerve impulses along certain nerve pathways. As a result, it relaxes blood vessels so that blood passes through them more easily. This helps to lower blood pressure.

Clonidine may also be used for other conditions as determined by your doctor.

Clonidine is available only with your doctor's prescription.

Before Using This Medicine

To decide on the best treatment for your medical problem, your doctor should be told:

—if you have ever had any unusual or allergic reaction to clonidine.

—if you are on a low-salt, low-sugar, or any other special diet, or if you are allergic to any substance, such as food, sulfites or other preservatives, or dyes. Most medicines contain more than their active ingredient. Your doctor, nurse, or pharmacist can help you avoid products that may cause a problem.

—if you are **pregnant** or if you may become pregnant. Studies have not been done in humans. Although clonidine has not been shown to cause birth defects in animals, it has been shown to cause toxic or harmful effects in the animal fetus, even at doses of only one-third the maximum human dose.

—if you are **breast-feeding**. Although clonidine passes into breast milk, it has not been shown to cause problems in nursing babies.

—if you have any of the following medical problems:
    Heart or blood vessel disease
    Irritated or scraped skin—with transdermal (skin patch) system only
    Kidney disease
    Mental depression (history of)
    Raynaud's syndrome
    Systemic lupus erythematosus (SLE)—with transdermal (skin patch) system only

—if you are taking **any** other prescription or nonprescription (OTC) medicine, especially one that contains:
    Beta-blockers (acebutolol [e.g., Sectral], atenolol [e.g., Tenormin], labetalol [e.g., Normodyne], metoprolol [e.g., Lopressor], nadolol [e.g., Corgard], oxprenolol [e.g., Trasicor], pindolol [e.g., Visken], propranolol [e.g., Inderal], sotalol [e.g., Sotacor], timolol [e.g., Blocadren])
    Tricyclic antidepressants (amitriptyline [e.g., Elavil], amoxapine [e.g., Asendin], clomipramine [e.g., Anafranil], desipramine [e.g., Pertofrane], doxepin [e.g., Sinequan], imipramine [e.g., Tofranil], nortriptyline [e.g., Aventyl], protriptyline [e.g., Vivactil], trimipramine [e.g., Surmontil])

Proper Use of This Medicine

For patients taking this medicine for high blood pressure:

• Importance of diet—When prescribing medicine for your condition, your doctor may also prescribe a personal diet for you. Such a diet may be low in sodium (salt). Most people eat much more sodium than they need and too much sodium in the diet may increase blood pressure. Some foods that contain large amounts of sodium are canned soup, pickles, ketchup, green and ripe olives, relish, frankfurters, soy sauce, and carbonated beverages. Your doctor may want you to limit the amounts of these and other high-sodium foods in your diet. High blood pressure medicine is usually more effective when such a diet is properly followed.

Also, it may be very important for you to go on a reducing diet. However, check with your doctor before changing your diet.

• Many patients who have high blood pressure will not notice any signs of the problem. In fact, many may feel normal. It is very important that you **take your medicine exactly as directed** and that you keep your appointments with your doctor even if you feel well.

• Remember that this medicine will not cure your high blood pressure but it does help control it. Therefore, you must continue to use it as directed if you expect to lower your blood pressure and keep it down. **You may have to take high blood pressure medicine for the rest of your life.** If high blood pressure is not treated, it can cause serious problems such as heart failure, blood vessel disease, stroke, or kidney disease.

For patients using the transdermal (stick-on patch) system:

• **Use this medicine exactly as directed by your doctor.** It will work only if applied correctly. **This medicine usually comes with patient instructions. Read them carefully before using.**

• Do not try to trim or cut the adhesive patch to adjust the dosage. Check with your doctor if you think the medicine is not working as it should.

• Apply the patch to a clean, dry area of skin on your upper arm or chest. Choose an area with little or no hair and free of scars, cuts, or irritation.

• The system should stay in place even during showering, bathing, or swimming. If the patch becomes loose, cover it with the extra adhesive overlay. Apply a new patch if the first one becomes too loose or falls off.

• Each dose is best applied to a different area of skin to prevent skin problems or other irritation.

To help you remember to use your medicine, try to get into the habit of using it at regular times. If you are taking the tablets, take them at the same time each day. If you are using the transdermal system, try to change it at the same time of day each week.

If you do miss a dose of this medicine, take it or use it as soon as possible. Then go back to your regular dosing schedule. **If you miss two or more doses of the tablets in a row or if you miss changing the transdermal patch for three or more days, check with your doctor right away.** If your body goes without this medicine for too long, your blood pressure may go up to a dangerously high level and some unpleasant effects may occur.

How to store this medicine:

- **Keep out of the reach of children.**

- Store away from heat and direct light.

- Do not store in the bathroom, near the kitchen sink, or in other damp places. Heat or moisture may cause the medicine to break down.

- Do not keep outdated medicine or medicine no longer needed. Be sure that any discarded medicine is out of the reach of children.

Precautions While Using This Medicine

It is important that your doctor check your progress at regular visits to make sure that this medicine is working properly.

Check with your doctor before you stop using this medicine. Your doctor may want you to reduce gradually the amount you are using before stopping completely.

Make sure that you have enough clonidine on hand to last through weekends, holidays, or vacations. You should not miss any doses. You may want to ask your doctor for another written prescription for clonidine to carry in your wallet or purse. You can then have it filled if you run out of medicine when you are away from home.

For patients taking this medicine for high blood pressure:

- **Do not take other medicines unless they have been discussed with your doctor.** This especially includes over-the-counter (nonprescription) medicines for appetite control, asthma, colds, cough, hay fever, or sinus problems, since they may tend to increase your blood pressure.

Clonidine will add to the effects of alcohol and other CNS depressants (medicines that slow down the nervous system, possibly causing drowsiness). Some examples of CNS depressants are antihistamines or medicine for hay fever, other allergies, or colds; sedatives, tranquilizers, or sleeping medicine; prescription pain medicine or narcotics; barbiturates; medicine for seizures; muscle relaxants; or anesthetics, including some dental anesthetics. **Check with your doctor before taking any of the above while you are using this medicine.**

Clonidine may cause some people to become drowsy or less alert than they are normally. This is more likely to happen when you begin to take it or when you increase the amount of medicine you are taking. **Make sure you know how you react to this medicine before you drive, use machines, or do other jobs that could be dangerous if you are not alert.**

Before having any kind of surgery (including dental surgery) or emergency treatment, **tell the physician or dentist in charge that you are using this medicine.**

Dizziness, lightheadedness, or fainting may occur, especially when you get up from a lying or sitting position. Getting up slowly may help but if the problem continues or gets worse, check with your doctor.

The dizziness, lightheadedness, or fainting is also more likely to occur if you drink alcohol, stand for long periods of time, exercise, or if the weather is hot. While you are taking clonidine, be careful in the amount of alcohol you drink. Also, use extra care during exercise or hot weather or if you must stand for long periods of time.

Clonidine may cause dryness of the mouth. For temporary relief, use sugarless candy or gum, melt bits of ice in your mouth, or use a saliva substitute. However, if dry mouth continues for more than 2 weeks, check with your physician or dentist. Continuing dryness of the mouth may increase the chance of dental disease, including tooth decay, gum disease, and fungus infections.

Side Effects of This Medicine

Along with its needed effects, a medicine may cause some unwanted effects. Although not all of these side effects may occur, if they do occur they may need medical attention.

Check with your doctor immediately if any of the following side effects occur:

Signs and symptoms of overdose

Difficulty in breathing
Dizziness (extreme) or faintness
Pinpoint pupils of eyes
Slow heartbeat
Unusual tiredness or weakness (extreme)

Check with your doctor as soon as possible if any of the following side effects occur:

More common—with transdermal system only

Itching or redness of skin

Less common

Darkening of skin—with transdermal system only
Mental depression
Swelling of feet and lower legs

Rare

Paleness or cold feeling in fingertips and toes
Vivid dreams or nightmares

Other side effects may occur that usually do not require medical attention. These side effects may go away during treatment as your body adjusts to the medicine. However, check with your doctor if any of the following side effects continue or are bothersome:

More common

Constipation
Dizziness
Drowsiness
Dry mouth
Unusual tiredness or weakness

Less common

Decreased sexual ability
Dizziness, lightheadedness, or fainting, especially when getting up from a lying or sitting position
Dry, itching, or burning eyes
Loss of appetite
Nausea or vomiting

Nervousness
Painful salivary glands
Trouble in sleeping

After you have been using this medicine for a while, it may cause unpleasant or even harmful effects if you stop taking it too suddenly. After you stop taking this medicine, **check with your doctor immediately** if any of the following occur:

Anxiety or tenseness
Chest pain
Fast or irregular heartbeat
Headache
Increased salivation
Nausea
Nervousness
Restlessness
Shaking or trembling of hands and fingers
Stomach cramps
Sweating
Trouble in sleeping
Vomiting

For elderly patients:

• Some medicines may affect older patients differently than they do younger adults. Dizziness or faintness may be more likely to occur in the elderly, who are more sensitive to the effects of clonidine. Check with your doctor if this continues or is bothersome. In addition, it is a good idea to check with your doctor or pharmacist if you notice any unusual effects while taking this medicine or if you think it is not working as it should.

Other side effects not listed above may also occur in some patients. If you notice any other effects, check with your doctor.

CLONIDINE AND CHLORTHALIDONE (Systemic)

A commonly used brand name in the U.S. and Canada is Combipres.

Generic name product may also be available in the U.S.

Clonidine (KLOE-ni-deen) and chlorthalidone (klor-THAL-i-done) combinations are used in the treatment of high blood pressure. High blood pressure adds to the workload of the heart and arteries. If it continues for a long time, the heart and arteries may not function properly. This can damage the blood vessels of the brain, heart, and kidneys resulting in a stroke, heart failure, or kidney failure. Hypertension may also increase the risk of heart attacks. These problems may be less likely to occur if blood pressure is controlled.

Clonidine works by controlling nerve impulses along certain body nerve pathways. As a result, it relaxes blood vessels so that blood passes through them more easily. The chlorthalidone in this combination is a diuretic (water pill) that helps reduce the amount of water in the body by increasing the flow of urine.

Clonidine and chlorthalidone combination is available only with your doctor's prescription.

Before Using This Medicine

To decide on the best treatment for your medical problem, your doctor should be told:

—if you have ever had any unusual or allergic reaction to clonidine, chlorthalidone, sulfonamides (sulfa drugs), or other thiazide diuretics (water pills).

—if you are on a low-salt, low-sugar, or any other special diet, or if you are allergic to any substance, such as foods, sulfites or other preservatives, or dyes. Most medicines contain more than their active ingredient. Your doctor, nurse, or pharmacist can help you avoid products that may cause a problem.

—if you are **pregnant** or if you may become pregnant. Studies with clonidine have not been done in humans. Although clonidine has not been shown to cause birth defects in animals, it has been shown to cause toxic or harmful effects in the fetus in animals even at doses of only one-third the maximum human dose. When chlorthalidone is used during pregnancy, it may cause side effects including jaundice, blood problems, and low potassium in the newborn infant.

—if you are **breast-feeding**. Although both clonidine and chlorthalidone pass into breast milk, they have not been shown to cause problems in nursing babies.

—if you have any of the following medical problems:

    Diabetes mellitus (sugar diabetes)
    Gout
    Heart or blood vessel disease
    Kidney disease
    Liver disease
    Lupus erythematosus (history of)
    Mental depression (history of)
    Pancreatitis (inflammation of the pancreas)
    Problems with veins

—if you are taking **any** other prescription or nonprescription (OTC) medicine, especially one that contains:

    Adrenocorticoids (cortisone-like medicines)
    Beta-blockers (acebutolol [e.g., Sectral], atenolol [e.g., Tenormin], labetalol [e.g., Normodyne], metoprolol [e.g., Lopressor], nadolol [e.g., Corgard], oxprenolol [e.g., Trasicor], pindolol [e.g., Visken], propranolol [e.g., Inderal], sotalol [e.g., Sotacor], timolol [e.g., Blocadren])
    Digitalis glycosides (heart medicine)
    Lithium (e.g., Lithane)
    Methenamine (e.g., Mandelamine)
    Tricyclic antidepressants (amitriptyline [e.g., Elavil], amoxapine [e.g., Asendin], clomipramine, desipramine [e.g., Pertofrane], doxepin [e.g., Sinequan], imipramine [e.g., Tofranil], nortriptyline [e.g., Aventyl], protriptyline [e.g., Vivactil], trimipramine [e.g., Surmontil])

Proper Use of This Medicine

This medicine may cause you to have an unusual feeling of tiredness when you begin to take it. You may also notice an increase in the amount of urine or in your frequency of urination. After taking the medicine for a while, these effects should lessen. In general, to keep the increase in urine from affecting your sleep:

• If you are to take a single dose a day, take it in the morning after breakfast.

• If you are to take more than one dose a day, take the last dose no later than 6 p.m., unless otherwise directed by your doctor.

However, it is best to plan your dose or doses according to a schedule that will least affect your personal activities and sleep. Ask your doctor, nurse, or pharmacist to help you plan the best time to take this medicine.

Importance of diet—When prescribing medicine for your condition, your doctor may also prescribe a personal diet for you. Such a diet may be low in sodium (salt). Most people eat much more sodium than they need and too much sodium in the diet may increase blood pressure. Some foods that contain large amounts of sodium are canned soup, pickles, ketchup, green and ripe olives, relish, frankfurters, soy sauce, and carbonated beverages. Your doctor may want you to limit the amounts of these and other high-sodium foods in your diet. High blood pressure medicine is usually more effective when such a diet is properly followed.

Also, it may be very important for you to go on a reducing diet. However, check with your doctor before changing your diet.

Many patients who have high blood pressure will not notice any signs of the problem. In fact, many may feel normal. It is very important that you **take your medicine exactly as directed** and that you keep your appointments with your doctor even if you feel well.

Remember that this medicine will not cure your high blood pressure but it does help control it. Therefore, you must continue to take it as directed if you expect to lower your blood pressure and keep it down. **You may have to take high blood pressure medicine for the rest of your life.** If high blood pressure is not treated, it can cause serious problems such as heart failure, blood vessel disease, stroke, or kidney disease.

To help you remember to take your medicine, try to get into the habit of taking it at the same time each day.

If you do miss a dose of this medicine, take it as soon as possible. Then go back to your regular dosing schedule. **If you miss two or more doses in a row, check with your doctor right away.** If your body goes without this medicine for too long, your blood pressure may go up to a dangerously high level.

How to store this medicine:

- **Keep out of the reach of children.**

- Store away from heat and direct light.

- Do not store in the bathroom, near the kitchen sink, or in other damp places. Heat or moisture may cause the medicine to break down.

- Do not keep outdated medicine or medicine no longer needed. Be sure that any discarded medicine is out of the reach of children.

Precautions While Using This Medicine

It is important that your doctor check your progress at regular visits to make sure that this medicine is working properly.

Check with your doctor before you stop taking this medicine. Your doctor may want you to reduce gradually the amount you are taking before stopping completely.

Make sure that you have enough medicine on hand to last through weekends, holidays, or vacations. You should not miss taking any doses. You may want to ask your doctor for another written prescription to carry in your wallet or purse. You can then have it filled if you run out of medicine when you are away from home.

Before having any kind of surgery (including dental surgery) or emergency treatment, **make sure the physician or dentist in charge knows that you are taking this medicine.**

Do not take other medicines unless they have been discussed with your doctor. This especially includes over-the-counter (nonprescription) medicines for appetite control, asthma, colds, cough, hay fever, or sinus problems, since they may tend to increase your blood pressure.

This medicine will add to the effects of alcohol and other CNS depressants (medicines that slow down the nervous system, possibly causing drowsiness). Some examples of CNS depressants are antihistamines or medicine for hay fever, other allergies, or colds; sedatives, tranquilizers, or sleeping medicine; prescription pain medicine or narcotics; barbiturates; medicine for seizures; muscle relaxants; or anesthetics, including some dental anesthetics. **Check with your doctor before taking any of the above while you are using this medicine.**

This medicine may cause some people to become drowsy or less alert than they are normally. This is more likely to happen when you begin to take it or when you increase the amount of medicine you are taking. **Make sure you know how you react to this medicine before you drive, use machines, or do other jobs that could be dangerous if you are not alert.**

Dizziness, lightheadedness, or fainting may occur, especially when you get up from a lying or sitting position. Getting up slowly may help but if the problem continues or gets worse, check with your doctor.

The dizziness, lightheadedness, or fainting is also more likely to occur if you drink alcohol, stand for long periods of time, exercise, or if the weather is hot. Drinking alcoholic beverages may also make the drowsiness worse. While you are taking this medicine, be careful in the amount of alcohol you drink. Also, use extra care during exercise or hot weather or if you must stand for long periods of time.

This medicine may cause a loss of potassium from your body.

- To help prevent this, your doctor may want you to:
    —eat or drink foods that have a high potassium content (for example, orange or other citrus fruit juices), or
    —take a potassium supplement, or

—take another medicine to help prevent the loss of the potassium in the first place.

• It is very important to follow these directions. Also, it is important not to change your diet on your own. This is more important if you are already on a special diet (as for diabetes), or if you are taking a potassium supplement or a medicine to reduce potassium loss. Extra potassium may not be necessary and, in some cases, too much potassium could be harmful.

Check with your doctor if you become sick and have severe or continuing vomiting or diarrhea. These problems may cause you to lose additional water and potassium.

For diabetic patients:

• Thiazide diuretics like chlorthalidone may raise blood sugar levels. While you are using this medicine, be especially careful in testing for sugar in your urine.

A few people who take this medicine may become more sensitive to sunlight than they are normally. When you first begin taking this medicine, avoid too much sun and do not use a sunlamp until you see how you react to the sun, especially if you tend to burn easily. If you have a severe reaction, check with your doctor.

This medicine may cause dryness of the mouth. For temporary relief, use sugarless candy or gum, melt bits of ice in your mouth, or use a saliva substitute. However, if dry mouth continues for more than 2 weeks, check with your physician or dentist. Continuing dryness of the mouth may increase the chance of dental disease, including tooth decay, gum disease, and fungus infections.

Side Effects of This Medicine

Along with its needed effects, a medicine may cause some unwanted effects. Although not all of these side effects may occur, if they do occur they may need medical attention.

Check with your doctor immediately if any of the following side effects occur:

Signs and symptoms of overdose
    Difficulty in breathing
    Dizziness (extreme) or faintness

Pinpoint pupils of eyes
Slow heartbeat
Unusual tiredness or weakness (extreme)

Check with your doctor as soon as possible if any of the following side effects occur, especially since some of them may mean that your body is losing too much potassium:

Signs and symptoms of too much potassium loss

Dryness of mouth
Increased thirst
Irregular heartbeats
Mood or mental changes
Muscle cramps or pain
Nausea or vomiting
Weak pulse

Rare

Joint, lower back or side, or stomach pain
Paleness or cold feeling in fingertips and toes
Skin rash or hives
Sore throat and fever
Stomach pain (severe) with nausea and vomiting
Unusual bleeding or bruising
Vivid dreams or nightmares
Yellow eyes or skin

Other side effects may occur that usually do not require medical attention. These side effects may go away during treatment as your body adjusts to the medicine. However, check with your doctor if any of the following side effects continue or are bothersome:

More common

Drowsiness

Less common

Constipation
Decreased sexual ability
Diarrhea
Dizziness or lightheadedness when getting up from a lying or sitting position
Dry, itching, or burning eyes
Increased sensitivity of skin to sunlight
Loss of appetite
Nervousness

Painful salivary glands
Trouble in sleeping
Upset stomach

After you have been using this medicine for a while, it may cause unpleasant or even harmful effects if you stop taking it too suddenly. After you stop taking this medicine, check with your doctor if any of the following occur:

Anxiety or tenseness
Chest pain
Fast or irregular heartbeat
Headache
Increased salivation
Nausea
Nervousness
Restlessness
Shaking or trembling of hands and fingers
Stomach cramps
Sweating
Trouble in sleeping
Vomiting

For elderly patients:

• Some medicines may affect older patients differently than they do younger adults. Dizziness or faintness may be more likely to occur in the elderly, who are more sensitive to the effects of clonidine and chlorthalidone. Check with your doctor if this continues or is bothersome. In addition, it is a good idea to check with your doctor or pharmacist if you notice any unusual effects while taking this medicine or if you think it is not working as it should.

Other side effects not listed above may also occur in some patients. If you notice any other effects, check with your doctor.

DIURETICS, LOOP (Systemic)

This information applies to the following medicines:

Bumetanide (byoo-MET-a-nide)
Ethacrynic acid (eth-a-KRIN-ik AS-id)
Furosemide (fur-OH-se-mide)

Some commonly used brand names are:

For Bumetanide†
In the U.S.
Bumex

For Ethacrynic Acid
In the U.S. and Canada
Edecrin

For Furosemide
In the U.S.
Lasix   Myrosemide

Generic name product may also be available.

In Canada
Apo-Furosemide   Lasix Special
Furoside   Novosemide
Lasix   Uritol

Generic name product may also be available.

---

†Not commercially available in Canada.

Loop diuretics are given to help reduce the amount of water in the body. They work by acting on the kidneys to increase the flow of urine.

Furosemide is also used to treat high blood pressure in those patients who are not helped by other medicines or in those patients who have kidney problems. High blood pressure adds to the workload of the heart and arteries. If it continues for a long time, the heart and arteries may not function properly. This can damage the blood vessels of the brain, heart, and kidneys, resulting in a stroke, heart failure, or kidney failure. High blood pressure may also increase the risk of heart attacks. These problems may be less likely to occur if blood pressure is controlled.

Loop diuretics may also be used for other conditions as determined by your doctor.

This medicine is available only with your doctor's prescription.

Before Using This Medicine

To decide on the best treatment for your medical problem, your doctor should be told:

—if you have ever had any unusual or allergic reaction to bumetanide, ethacrynic acid, furosemide, sulfonamides (sulfa drugs), or thiazide diuretics (water pills).

—if you are on a low-salt, low-sugar, or any other special diet, or if you are allergic to any substance, such as foods, sulfites or other preservatives, or dyes. Most medicines contain more than their active ingredient, and many liquid medicines contain alcohol. Your doctor, nurse, or pharmacist can help you avoid products that may cause a problem.

—if you are **pregnant** or if you may become pregnant. Studies have not been done in humans. However, studies in animals have shown this medicine to cause harmful effects. Also, ethacrynic acid causes birth defects in animals.

In general, diuretics are not useful for normal swelling of feet and hands that occurs during pregnancy. Diuretics should not be taken during pregnancy unless recommended by your doctor.

—if you are **breast-feeding**. This medicine has not been shown to cause problems in nursing babies. Furosemide passes into breast milk; it is not known whether bumetanide or ethacrynic acid passes into breast milk.

—if you have any of the following medical problems:
Diabetes mellitus (sugar diabetes)
Diarrhea
Gout
Hearing problems
Kidney disease (severe)
Liver disease
Lupus erythematosus (history of)
Pancreas disease

—if you have recently had a heart attack.

—if you are taking **any** other prescription or nonprescription (OTC) medicine, especially one that contains:
Adrenocorticoids (cortisone-like medicines)
Amphotericin B by injection (e.g., Fungizone)

Anticoagulants (blood thinners)
Captopril (e.g., Capoten)
Carmustine (e.g., BiCNU)
Cisplatin (e.g., Platinol)
Cyclosporine (e.g., Sandimmune)
Deferoxamine (e.g., Desferal) (with long-term use)
Enalapril (e.g., Vasotec)
Gold salts
Lithium (e.g., Lithane)
Medicine for infection
Medicine for inflammation or pain, except narcotics
Methotrexate (e.g., Mexate)
Penicillamine (e.g., Cuprimine)
Plicamycin (e.g., Mithracin)
Streptozocin (e.g., Zanosar)

—if you regularly take large amounts of combination pain medicine containing acetaminophen and aspirin or other salicylates.

Proper Use of This Medicine

This medicine may cause you to have an unusual feeling of tiredness when you begin to take it. You may also notice an increase in the amount of urine or in your frequency of urination. After taking the medicine for a while, these effects should lessen. To keep the increase in urine from affecting your nighttime sleep:

• If you are to take a single dose a day, take it in the morning after breakfast.

• If you are to take more than one dose a day, take the last dose no later than 6 p.m., unless otherwise directed by your doctor.

However, it is best to plan your dose or doses according to a schedule that will least affect your personal activities and sleep. Ask your doctor, nurse, or pharmacist to help you plan the best time to take this medicine.

To help you remember to take your medicine, try to get into the habit of taking it at the same time each day.

For patients taking the oral liquid form of furosemide:

• This medicine is to be taken by mouth even if it comes in a dropper bottle. If this medicine does not come in a dropper bottle, use a specially marked measuring spoon or other device to measure each dose accurately, since the average household teaspoon may not hold the right amount of liquid.

For patients taking this medicine for high blood pressure:

• Importance of diet—When prescribing medicine for your condition, your doctor may prescribe a personal diet for you. Such a diet may be low in sodium (salt). Most people eat much more sodium than they need and too much sodium in the diet may increase blood pressure. Some foods that contain large amounts of sodium are canned soup, pickles, ketchup, green and ripe olives, relish, frankfurters, soy sauce, and carbonated beverages. Your doctor may want you to limit the amounts of these and other high-sodium foods in your diet. High blood pressure medicine is usually more effective when such a diet is properly followed.

Also, it may be very important for you to go on a reducing diet. However, check with your doctor before changing your diet.

• Many patients who have high blood pressure will not notice any signs of the problem. In fact, many may feel normal. It is very important that you **take your medicine exactly as directed** and that you keep your appointments with your doctor even if you feel well.

• Remember that this medicine will not cure your high blood pressure but it does help control it. Therefore, you must continue to take it as directed if you expect to lower your blood pressure and keep it down. **You may have to take high blood pressure medicine for the rest of your life.** If high blood pressure is not treated, it can cause serious problems such as heart failure, blood vessel disease, stroke, or kidney disease.

If this medicine upsets your stomach, it may be taken with meals or milk. If stomach upset (nausea, vomiting, or stomach pain) continues or gets worse, or if you suddenly get severe diarrhea, check with your doctor.

If you miss a dose of this medicine, take it as soon as possible. However, if it is almost time for your next dose, skip the

missed dose and go back to your regular dosing schedule. Do not double doses.

How to store this medicine:

- **Keep out of the reach of children.**

- Store away from heat and direct light.

- Do not store in the bathroom, near the kitchen sink, or in other damp places. Heat or moisture may cause the medicine to break down.

- Keep the oral liquid form of this medicine from freezing.

- Do not keep outdated medicine or medicine no longer needed. Be sure that any discarded medicine is out of the reach of children.

Precautions While Using This Medicine

It is important that your doctor check your progress at regular visits to make sure that this medicine is working properly.

This medicine may cause a loss of potassium from your body.

- To help prevent this, your doctor may want you to:

  —eat or drink foods that have a high potassium content (for example, orange or other citrus fruit juices), or

  —take a potassium supplement, or

  —take another medicine to help prevent the loss of the potassium in the first place.

- It is very important to follow these directions. Also, it is important not to change your diet on your own. This is more important if you are already on a special diet (as for diabetes), or if you are taking a potassium supplement or a medicine to reduce potassium loss. Extra potassium may not be necessary and, in some cases, too much potassium could be harmful.

To prevent the loss of too much water and potassium, tell your doctor if you become sick, especially with severe or continuing nausea and vomiting or diarrhea.

Before having any kind of surgery (including dental surgery) or emergency treatment, make sure the physician or dentist in charge knows that you are taking this medicine.

Dizziness, lightheadedness, or fainting may occur, especially when you get up from a lying or sitting position. This is more likely to occur in the morning. **Getting up slowly may help,** but if the problem continues or gets worse, check with your doctor.

The dizziness, lightheadedness, or fainting is also more likely to occur if you drink alcohol, stand for long periods of time, or exercise, or if the weather is hot. **While you are taking this medicine, be careful of the amount of alcohol you drink. Also, use extra care during exercise or hot weather or if you must stand for long periods of time.**

For diabetic patients:

• This medicine may affect blood sugar levels. While you are using this medicine, be especially careful in testing for sugar in your blood or urine.

For patients taking this medicine for high blood pressure:

• **Do not take other medicines unless they have been discussed with your doctor.** This especially includes over-the-counter (nonprescription) medicines for appetite control, asthma, colds, cough, hay fever, or sinus problems, since they may tend to increase your blood pressure.

For patients taking furosemide:

• Some people who take this medicine may become more sensitive to sunlight than they are normally. When you first begin taking this medicine, avoid too much sun and do not use a sunlamp until you see how you react to the sun, especially if you tend to burn easily. If you have a severe reaction, check with your doctor.

Side Effects of This Medicine

Along with its needed effects, a medicine may cause some unwanted effects. Although not all of these side effects may occur, if they do occur they may need medical attention.

Check with your doctor as soon as possible if any of the following side effects occur:

Rare

Black tarry stools—for ethacrynic acid injection only
Blood in urine—for ethacrynic acid injection only
Joint, lower back or side, or stomach pain
Ringing or buzzing in ears or any loss of hearing—more common with ethacrynic acid
Skin rash or hives
Sore throat and fever
Stomach pain (severe) with nausea and vomiting
Unusual bleeding or bruising
Yellow eyes or skin
Yellow vision—for furosemide only

Signs and symptoms of too much potassium loss

Dryness of mouth
Increased thirst
Irregular heartbeats
Mood or mental changes
Muscle cramps or pain
Nausea or vomiting
Unusual tiredness or weakness
Weak pulse

Other side effects may occur that usually do not require medical attention. These side effects may go away during treatment as your body adjusts to the medicine. However, check with your doctor if any of the following side effects continue or are bothersome:

More common

Dizziness or lightheadedness when getting up from a lying or sitting position

Less common or rare

Blurred vision
Chest pain—with bumetanide only
Confusion—with ethacrynic acid only
Diarrhea—more common with ethacrynic acid
Headache
Increased sensitivity of skin to sunlight—with furosemide only
Loss of appetite—more common with ethacrynic acid
Nervousness—with ethacrynic acid only
Premature ejaculation or difficulty in keeping an erection—with bumetanide only

Redness or pain at the place of injection
Stomach cramps or pain

For elderly patients:

• Some medicines may affect older patients differently than they do younger adults. Dizziness, light-headedness, or signs of too much potassium loss may be more likely to occur in the elderly, who are more sensitive to the effects of this medicine. Check with your doctor if this occurs. In addition, it is a good idea to check with your doctor or pharmacist if you notice any unusual effects while taking this medicine or if you think it is not working as it should.

Other side effects not listed above may also occur in some patients. If you notice any other effects, check with your doctor.

DIURETICS, POTASSIUM-SPARING
(Systemic)

This information applies to the following medicines:

Amiloride (a-MILL-oh-ride)
Spironolactone (speer-on-oh-LAK-tone)
Triamterene (trye-AM-ter-een)

Some commonly used brand names are:

For Amiloride
In the U.S.
Midamor

Generic name product may also be available.

In Canada
Midamor

For Spironolactone
In the U.S.
Aldactone

Generic name product may also be available.

In Canada
Aldactone   Sincomen
Novospiroton

For Triamterene
In the U.S. and Canada
Dyrenium

Potassium-sparing diuretics are commonly taken by mouth to help reduce the amount of water in the body. Unlike some other diuretics, these medicines do not cause your body to lose potassium.

Amiloride and spironolactone are also used to treat high blood pressure. High blood pressure adds to the workload of the heart and arteries. If it continues for a long time, the heart and arteries may not function properly. This can damage the blood vessels of the brain, heart, and kidneys resulting in a stroke, heart failure, or kidney failure. High blood pressure may also increase the risk of heart attacks. These problems may be less likely to occur if blood pressure is controlled.

Spironolactone is also used to help increase the amount of potassium in the body when it is getting too low.

Potassium-sparing diuretics help to reduce the amount of water in the body by acting on the kidneys to increase the flow of urine. This also helps to lower blood pressure.

These medicines can also be used for other conditions as determined by your doctor.

Potassium-sparing diuretics are available only with your doctor's prescription.

Before Using This Medicine

To decide on the best treatment for your medical problem, your doctor should be told:

—if you have ever had any unusual or allergic reaction to amiloride, spironolactone, or triamterene.

—if you are on a low-salt, low-sugar, or any other special diet, or if you are allergic to any substance, such as foods, sulfites or other preservatives, or dyes. Most medicines contain more than their active ingredient. Your doctor, nurse, or pharmacist can help you avoid products that may cause a problem.

—if you are **pregnant** or if you may become pregnant. Studies have not been done in humans. However, this medicine has not been shown to cause birth defects or other problems in animals.

In general, diuretics are not useful for normal swelling of feet and hands that occurs during pregnancy. Diuretics should not be taken during pregnancy unless recommended by your doctor.

—if you are **breast-feeding**. Although spironolactone and triamterene may pass into breast milk, these medicines have not been shown to cause problems in nursing babies. It is not known whether amiloride passes into breast milk.

—if you have any of the following medical problems:
    Diabetes mellitus (sugar diabetes)
    Gout (triamterene only)
    Kidney disease
    Kidney stones (history of; triamterene only)
    Liver disease
    Menstrual problems or breast enlargement (spironolactone only)

—if you are taking **any** other prescription or nonprescription (OTC) medicine, especially one that contains:
    Captopril (e.g., Capoten)
    Cyclosporine (e.g., Sandimmune)

Enalapril (e.g., Vasotec)
Lisinopril (e.g., Prinivil, Zestril)
Lithium (e.g., Lithane)
Potassium-containing medicines or supplements

Proper Use of This Medicine

This medicine may cause you to have an unusual feeling of tiredness when you begin to take it. You may also notice an increase in the amount of urine or in your frequency of urination. After taking the medicine for a while, these effects should lessen. In general, in order to keep the increase in urine from affecting your nighttime sleep:

• If you are to take a single dose a day, take it in the morning after breakfast.

• If you are to take more than one dose a day, take the last dose no later than 6 p.m., unless otherwise directed by your doctor.

However, it is best to plan your dose or doses according to a schedule that will least affect your personal activities and sleep. Ask your doctor, nurse, or pharmacist to help you plan the best time to take this medicine.

To help you remember to take your medicine, try to get into the habit of taking it at the same time each day.

If this medicine upsets your stomach, it may be taken with meals or milk. If stomach upset (nausea, vomiting, stomach pain or cramps) continues, check with your doctor.

For patients taking this medicine for high blood pressure:
• Importance of diet—When prescribing medicine for your condition, your doctor may also prescribe a personal diet for you. Such a diet may be low in sodium (salt). Most people eat much more sodium than they need and too much sodium in the diet may increase blood pressure. Some foods that contain large amounts of sodium are canned soup, pickles, ketchup, green and ripe olives, relish, frankfurters, soy sauce, and carbonated beverages. Your doctor may want you to limit the amounts of these and other high-sodium foods in your diet. High blood pressure medicine is usually more effective when such a diet is properly followed.

Also, it may be very important for you to go on a reducing diet. However, check with your doctor before changing your diet.

• Many patients who have high blood pressure will not notice any signs of the problem. In fact, many may feel normal. It is very important that you **take your medicine exactly as directed** and that you keep your appointments with your doctor even if you feel well.

• Remember that this medicine will not cure your high blood pressure but it does help control it. Therefore, you must continue to take it as directed if you expect to lower your blood pressure and keep it down. **You may have to take high blood pressure medicine for the rest of your life.** If high blood pressure is not treated, it can cause serious problems such as heart failure, blood vessel disease, stroke, or kidney disease.

If you miss a dose of this medicine, take it as soon as possible. However, if it is almost time for your next dose, skip the missed dose and go back to your regular dosing schedule. Do not double doses.

How to store this medicine:

• **Keep out of the reach of children.**

• Store away from heat and direct light.

• Do not store in the bathroom, near the kitchen sink, or in other damp places. Heat or moisture may cause the medicine to break down.

• Do not keep outdated medicine or medicine no longer needed. Be sure that any discarded medicine is out of the reach of children.

Precautions While Using This Medicine

It is important that your doctor check your progress at regular visits to make sure that this medicine is working properly.

This medicine does not cause a loss of potassium from your body as some other diuretics (water pills) do. Therefore, it is not necessary for you to get extra potassium in your diet, and too much potassium could even be harmful. Since salt substitutes and low-salt milk may contain potassium, do not use them unless told to do so by your doctor.

Check with your doctor if you become sick and have severe or continuing nausea, vomiting, or diarrhea. These problems may cause you to lose additional water, which could be harmful, or to lose potassium, which could lessen the medicine's helpful effects.

Before having any kind of surgery (including dental surgery) or emergency treatment, tell the physician or dentist in charge that you are taking this medicine.

For patients taking this medicine for high blood pressure:

• **Do not take other medicines unless they have been discussed with your doctor.** This especially includes over-the-counter (nonprescription) medicines for appetite control, asthma, colds, cough, hay fever, or sinus problems, since they may tend to increase your blood pressure.

For patients taking triamterene:

• Diabetics—This medicine may raise blood sugar levels. While you are using triamterene, be especially careful in testing for sugar in your urine. If you have any questions about this, check with your doctor.

• A few people who take this medicine may become more sensitive to sunlight than they are normally. When you first begin taking triamterene, avoid too much sun and do not use a sunlamp until you see how you react to the sun, especially if you tend to burn easily. If you have a severe reaction, check with your doctor.

Tell the doctor in charge that you are taking this medicine before you have any medical tests. The results of some tests may be affected by this medicine.

Side Effects of This Medicine

In rats, spironolactone has been found to increase the risk of tumors. It is not known if spironolactone increases the chance of tumors in humans.

Along with its needed effects, a medicine may cause some unwanted effects. Although not all of these side effects may occur, if they do occur they may need medical attention.

Check with your doctor as soon as possible if any of the following side effects occur:

Rare

Shortness of breath
Skin rash or itching

Signs and symptoms of too much potassium

Confusion
Irregular heartbeat
Nervousness
Numbness or tingling in hands, feet, or lips
Shortness of breath or difficult breathing
Unusual tiredness or weakness
Weakness or heaviness of legs

Reported for triamterene only (rare)

Bright red tongue
Burning, inflamed feeling in tongue
Cracked corners of mouth
Lower back or side pain (severe)
Sore throat and fever
Unusual bleeding or bruising
Weakness

For elderly patients:

• Some medicines may affect older patients differently than they do younger adults. Signs and symptoms of too much potassium are more likely to occur in the elderly, who are more sensitive to the effects of this medicine. Check with your doctor if this occurs. In addition, it is a good idea to check with your doctor or pharmacist if you notice any unusual effects while taking this medicine or if you think it is not working as it should.

Other side effects may occur that usually do not require medical attention. These side effects may go away during treatment as your body adjusts to the medicine.

However, check with your doctor if any of the following side effects continue or are bothersome:

More common (less common with amiloride and triamterene)

Nausea and vomiting
Stomach cramps and diarrhea

Less common

Dizziness
Headache

Signs and symptoms of too little sodium

Drowsiness
Dryness of mouth
Increased thirst
Lack of energy

Reported for amiloride and spironolactone only (less common)

Constipation
Decreased sexual ability
Muscle cramps

Reported for spironolactone only (less common)

Breast tenderness in females
Clumsiness
Deepening of voice in females
Enlargement of breasts in males
Inability to have or keep an erection
Increased hair growth in females
Irregular menstrual periods
Sweating

Reported for triamterene only (less common)

Increased sensitivity of skin to sunlight

For male patients:

• Spironolactone sometimes causes enlarged breasts in males, especially when they take large doses of it for a long time. Breasts usually decrease in size gradually over several months after this medicine is stopped. If you have any questions about this, check with your doctor.

Other side effects not listed above may also occur in some patients. If you notice any other effects, check with your doctor.

DIURETICS, POTASSIUM-SPARING, AND HYDROCHLOROTHIAZIDE (Systemic)

This information applies to the following medicines:

Amiloride (a-MILL-oh-ride) and Hydrochlorothiazide (hye-droe-klor-oh-THYE-a-zide)

Spironolactone (speer-on-oh-LAK-tone) and Hydrochlorothiazide

Triamterene (trye-AM-ter-een) and Hydrochlorothiazide

Some commonly used brand names are:

For Amiloride and Hydrochlorothiazide
In the U.S.

Moduretic

Generic name product may also be available.

In Canada

Moduret

For Spironolactone and Hydrochlorothiazide
In the U.S.

Aldactazide

Spirozide

Generic name product may also be available.

In Canada

Aldactazide

Novospirozine

For Triamterene and Hydrochlorothiazide
In the U.S.

Dyazide

Maxzide

Generic name product may also be available.

In Canada

Apo-Triazide   Novotriamzide

Dyazide

This medicine is a combination of two diuretics (water pills). It is commonly taken by mouth to help reduce the amount of water in the body.

This combination is also used to treat high blood pressure. High blood pressure adds to the workload of the heart and arteries. If it continues for a long time, the heart and arteries may not function properly. This can damage the blood vessels of the brain, heart, and kidneys, resulting in a stroke, heart failure, or kidney failure. High blood pressure may also increase the risk of heart attacks. These problems may be less likely to occur if blood pressure is controlled.

Diuretics help to reduce the amount of water in the body by acting on the kidneys to increase the flow of urine. This also helps to lower blood pressure.

This combination is also used to treat problems caused by too little potassium in the body.

This medicine is available only with your doctor's prescription.

Before Using This Medicine

To decide on the best treatment for your medical problem, your doctor should be told:

—if you have ever had any unusual or allergic reaction to amiloride, spironolactone, triamterene, sulfonamides (sulfa drugs), bumetanide, furosemide, acetazolamide, dichlorphenamide, methazolamide, or to hydrochlorothiazide or any of the other thiazide diuretics.

—if you are on a low-salt, low-sugar, or any other special diet, or if you are allergic to any substance, such as foods, sulfites or other preservatives, or dyes. Most medicines contain more than their active ingredient. Your doctor, nurse, or pharmacist can help you avoid products that may cause a problem.

—if you are **pregnant** or if you may become pregnant. When hydrochlorothiazide is used during pregnancy, it may cause side effects including jaundice, blood problems, and low potassium in the newborn infant. In addition, although this medicine has not been shown to cause birth defects, the chance always exists.

In general, diuretics are not useful for normal swelling of feet and hands that occurs during pregnancy. They should not be taken during pregnancy unless recommended by your doctor.

—if you are **breast-feeding**. Although spironolactone, triamterene, and hydrochlorothiazide may pass into breast milk, they have not been shown to cause problems in nursing babies. It is not known whether amiloride passes into breast milk.

—if you have any of the following medical problems:
    Diabetes mellitus (sugar diabetes)
    Gout (history of)

Kidney disease
Kidney stones (history of—triamterene only)
Liver disease
Lupus erythematosus (history of)
Menstrual problems or breast enlargement (spironolactone only)
Pancreatitis (inflammation of pancreas)

—if you are taking **any** other prescription or nonprescription (OTC) medicine, especially one that contains:

Adrenocorticoids (cortisone-like medicine)
Captopril (e.g., Capoten)
Cyclosporine (e.g., Sandimmune)
Digitalis glycosides (heart medicine)
Enalapril (e.g., Vasotec)
Lisinopril (e.g., Prinivil, Zestril)
Lithium (e.g., Lithane)
Methenamine (e.g., Mandelamine)
Other diuretics (water pills) or antihypertensives (high blood pressure medicine)
Potassium-containing medicines or supplements

Proper Use of This Medicine

This medicine may cause you to have an unusual feeling of tiredness when you begin to take it. You may also notice an increase in the amount of urine or in your frequency of urination. After you have taken the medicine for a while, these effects should lessen. In general, to keep the increase in urine from affecting your nighttime sleep:

• If you are to take a single dose a day, take it in the morning after breakfast.

• If you are to take more than one dose a day, take the last dose no later than 6 p.m., unless otherwise directed by your doctor.

However, it is best to plan your dose or doses according to a schedule that will least affect your personal activities and sleep. Ask your doctor, nurse, or pharmacist to help you plan the best time to take this medicine.

To help you remember to take your medicine, try to get into the habit of taking it at the same time each day.

If this medicine upsets your stomach, it may be taken with meals or milk. If stomach upset (nausea, vomiting, stomach pain, or cramps) continues, check with your doctor.

For patients taking this medicine for high blood pressure:

• Importance of diet—When prescribing medicine for your condition, your doctor may also prescribe a personal diet for you. Such a diet may be low in sodium (salt). Most people eat much more sodium than they need and too much sodium in the diet may increase blood pressure. Some foods that contain large amounts of sodium are canned soup, pickles, ketchup, green and ripe olives, relish, frankfurters, soy sauce, and carbonated beverages. Your doctor may want you to limit the amounts of these and other high-sodium foods in your diet. High blood pressure medicine is usually more effective when such a diet is properly followed.

However, some foods low in sodium, as well as some salt substitutes, are high in potassium. If they are used together with this medicine, they may lead to too much potassium in the body. Discuss with your doctor what low-sodium foods you may use.

Also, it may be very important for you to go on a reducing diet. However, check with your doctor before changing your diet.

• Many patients who have high blood pressure will not notice any signs of the problem. In fact, many may feel normal. It is very important that you **take your medicine exactly as directed** and that you keep your appointments with your doctor even if you feel well.

• Remember that this medicine will not cure your high blood pressure but it does help control it. Therefore, you must continue to take it as directed if you expect to lower your blood pressure and keep it down. **You may have to take high blood pressure medicine for the rest of your life.** If high blood pressure is not treated, it can cause serious problems such as heart failure, blood vessel disease, stroke, or kidney disease.

If you miss a dose of this medicine, take it as soon as possible. However, if it is almost time for your next dose, skip the

missed dose and go back to your regular dosing schedule.
Do not double doses.

How to store this medicine:

- **Keep out of the reach of children.**

- Store away from heat and direct light.

- Do not store in the bathroom, near the kitchen sink, or
in other damp places. Heat or moisture may cause the
medicine to break down.

- Do not keep outdated medicine or medicine no longer
needed. Be sure that any discarded medicine is out of the
reach of children.

Precautions While Using This Medicine

It is important that your doctor check your progress at regular visits to make sure that this medicine is working
properly.

**This medicine may cause a loss or increase of potassium in
your body. Your doctor may have special instructions about
whether or not you need to eat or drink foods or beverages
that have a high potassium content (for example, orange
or other citrus fruit juices), taking a potassium supplement, or using salt substitutes.** Since too much potassium
can be harmful, it is important not to change your diet
on your own. Tell your doctor if you are already on a
special diet (as for diabetes). Since salt substitutes and
low-salt milk may contain potassium, do not use them
unless told to do so by your doctor. Check with your
doctor, nurse, or pharmacist if you need a list of foods
that are high in potassium or if you have any questions.

Check with your doctor if you become sick and have severe
or continuing vomiting or diarrhea. These problems may
cause you to lose additional water and potassium and lead
to low blood pressure.

For diabetic patients:

- Hydrochlorothiazide (contained in this combination
medicine) may raise blood sugar levels. While you are
taking this medicine, be especially careful in testing for
sugar in your blood or urine.

A few people who take this medicine may become more sensitive to sunlight than they are normally. When you first begin taking this medicine, avoid too much sun and do not use a sunlamp until you see how you react to the sun, especially if you tend to burn easily. If you have a severe reaction, check with your doctor.

Before having any kind of surgery (including dental surgery) or emergency treatment, tell the physician or dentist in charge that you are taking this medicine.

For patients taking triamterene and hydrochlorothiazide combination:

• Do not change brands of triamterene and hydrochlorothiazide without first checking with your doctor. Different products may not work the same way. If you refill your medicine and it looks different, check with your pharmacist.

For patients taking this medicine for high blood pressure:

• **Do not take other medicines unless they have been discussed with your doctor.** This especially includes over-the-counter (nonprescription) medicines for appetite control, asthma, colds, cough, hay fever, or sinus problems, since they may tend to increase your blood pressure.

Tell the doctor in charge that you are taking this medicine before you have any medical tests. The results of some tests may be affected by this medicine.

Side Effects of This Medicine

In rats, spironolactone has been found to increase the risk of development of tumors. However, the doses given were many times the dose of spironolactone given to humans. It is not known whether spironolactone causes tumors in humans.

Along with its needed effects, a medicine may cause some unwanted effects. Although not all of these side effects may occur, if they do occur they may need medical attention.

Check with your doctor as soon as possible if any of the
following side effects occur:

Rare

Joint, lower back or side, or stomach pain
Skin rash or hives
Sore throat and fever
Stomach pain (severe) with nausea and vomiting
Unusual bleeding or bruising
Yellow eyes or skin

Signs and symptoms of changes in potassium

Dryness of mouth
Increased thirst
Irregular heartbeats
Mood or mental changes
Muscle cramps or pain
Numbness or tingling in hands, feet, or lips
Shortness of breath or difficulty breathing
Unusual tiredness or weakness
Weak pulse

Reported for triamterene only (rare)

Bright red tongue
Burning, inflamed feeling in tongue
Cracked corners of mouth

Other side effects may occur that usually do not require
medical attention. These side effects may go away
during treatment as your body adjusts to the medicine.
However, check with your doctor if any of the following side effects continue or are bothersome:

More common (less common with triamterene)

Loss of appetite
Nausea and vomiting
Stomach cramps and diarrhea
Upset stomach

Less common

Decreased sexual ability
Dizziness or lightheadedness when getting up from a lying
or sitting position
Headache (more common with amiloride)
Increased sensitivity of skin to sunlight

Reported for amiloride and triamterene only (less common)

Constipation

Reported for spironolactone only (less common)

Breast tenderness in females
Clumsiness
Deepening of voice in females
Enlargement of breasts in males
Increased hair growth in females
Irregular menstrual periods
Sweating

For elderly patients:

• Some medicines may affect older patients differently than they do younger adults. Dizziness or light-headedness and signs and symptoms of too much potassium loss may be more likely to occur in the elderly, who are more sensitive to the effects of this medicine. Check with your doctor if this occurs. In addition, it is a good idea to check with your doctor or pharmacist if you notice any unusual effects while you are taking this medicine or if you think it is not working as it should.

Spironolactone sometimes causes enlarged breasts in males, especially when they take large doses of it for a long time. Breasts usually decrease in size gradually over several months after this medicine is stopped. If you have any questions about this, check with your doctor.

Other side effects not listed above may also occur in some patients. If you notice any other effects, check with your doctor.

DIURETICS, THIAZIDE (Systemic)

This information applies to the following medicines:

Bendroflumethiazide (ben-droe-floo-meth-EYE-a-zide)
Benzthiazide (benz-THYE-a-zide)
Chlorothiazide (klor-oh-THYE-a-zide)
Chlorthalidone (klor-THAL-i-doan)
Cyclothiazide (sye-kloe-THYE-a-zide)
Hydrochlorothiazide (hye-droe-klor-oh-THYE-a-zide)
Hydroflumethiazide (hye-droe-floo-meth-EYE-a-zide)
Methyclothiazide (meth-ee-kloe-THYE-a-zide)
Metolazone (me-TOLE-a-zone)
Polythiazide (pol-i-THYE-a-zide)
Quinethazone (kwin-ETH-a-zone)
Trichlormethiazide (trye-klor-meth-EYE-a-zide)

Some commonly used brand names are:

For Bendroflumethiazide
In the U.S. and Canada
    Naturetin

For Benzthiazide†
In the U.S.
    Aquatag   Hydrex
    Exna

    Generic name product may also be available.

For Chlorothiazide†
In the U.S.
    Diuril

    Generic name product may also be available.

For Chlorthalidone
In the U.S.
    Hygroton
    Thalitone

    Generic name product may also be available.

In Canada
    Apo-Chlorthalidone   Novothalidone
    Hygroton   Uridon

    Generic name product may also be available.

Another commonly used name is chlortalidone.

For Cyclothiazide†
In the U.S.
    Anhydron
    Fluidil

For Hydrochlorothiazide
In the U.S.

Esidrix	Oretic
HydroDIURIL	Thiuretic
Mictrin	

Generic name product may also be available.

In Canada

Apo-Hydro	Neo-Codema
Diuchlor H	Novohydrazide
HydroDIURIL	Urozide
Natrimax	

Generic name product may also be available.

For Hydroflumethiazide†
In the U.S.
Diucardin
Saluron

Generic name product may also be available.

For Methyclothiazide
In the U.S.
Aquatensen
Enduron

Generic name product may also be available.

In Canada
Duretic

For Metolazone
In the U.S.

Diulo	Zaroxolyn
Microx	

In Canada
Zaroxolyn

For Polythiazide†
In the U.S.
Renese

For Quinethazone†
In the U.S.
Hydromox

For Trichlormethiazide†
In the U.S.
Metahydrin
Naqua

Generic name product may also be available.

---

†Not commercially available in Canada.

Thiazide or thiazide-like diuretics are commonly used to treat high blood pressure. High blood pressure adds to the workload of the heart and arteries. If it continues for a long time, the heart and arteries may not function properly. This can damage the blood vessels of the brain, heart, and kidneys, resulting in a stroke, heart failure, or kidney failure. High blood pressure may also increase the risk of heart attacks. These problems may be less likely to occur if blood pressure is controlled.

Thiazide diuretics are also used to help reduce the amount of water in the body by increasing the flow of urine. They may also be used for other conditions as determined by your doctor.

Thiazide diuretics are available only with your doctor's prescription.

Before Using This Medicine

To decide on the best treatment for your medical problem, your doctor should be told:

—if you have ever had any unusual or allergic reaction to sulfonamides (sulfa drugs) or any of the thiazide diuretics.

—if you are on a low-salt, low-sugar, or any other special diet, or if you are allergic to any substance, such as foods, sulfites or other preservatives, or dyes. Most medicines contain more than their active ingredient, and many liquid medicines contain alcohol. Your doctor, nurse, or pharmacist can help you avoid products that may cause a problem.

—if you are **pregnant** or if you may become pregnant. When this medicine is used during pregnancy, it may cause side effects including jaundice, blood problems, and low potassium in the newborn infant. In addition, although this medicine has not been shown to cause birth defects or other problems in animals, studies have not been done in humans.

In general, diuretics are not useful for normal swelling of feet and hands that occurs during pregnancy. They should not be taken during pregnancy unless recommended by your doctor.

—if you are **breast-feeding**. Although thiazide diuretics pass into breast milk, they have not been shown to cause problems in nursing babies.

—if you have any of the following medical problems:
Diabetes mellitus (sugar diabetes)
Gout (history of)
Kidney disease (severe)
Liver disease
Lupus erythematosus (history of)
Pancreatitis (inflammation of the pancreas)

—if you are taking or using **any** other prescription or nonprescription (OTC) medicine, especially one that contains:
Adrenocorticoids (cortisone-like medicines)
Digitalis glycosides (heart medicine)
Lithium (e.g., Lithane)
Methenamine (e.g., Mandelamine)

Proper Use of This Medicine

This medicine may cause you to have an unusual feeling of tiredness when you begin to take it. You may also notice an increase in the amount of urine or in your frequency of urination. After you have taken the medicine for a while, these effects should lessen. To keep the increase in urine from affecting your nighttime sleep:

• If you are to take a single dose a day, take it in the morning after breakfast.

• If you are to take more than one dose a day, take the last dose no later than 6 p.m., unless otherwise directed by your doctor.

However, it is best to plan your dose or doses according to a schedule that will least affect your personal activities and sleep. Ask your doctor, nurse, or pharmacist to help you plan the best time to take this medicine.

To help you remember to take your medicine, try to get into the habit of taking it at the same time each day.

For patients taking this medicine for high blood pressure:
• Importance of diet—When prescribing medicine for your condition, your doctor may also prescribe a personal diet for you. Such a diet may be low in sodium (salt).

Most people eat much more sodium than they need and too much sodium in the diet may increase blood pressure. Some foods that contain large amounts of sodium are canned soup, pickles, ketchup, green and ripe olives, relish, frankfurters, soy sauce, and carbonated beverages. Your doctor may want you to limit the amounts of these and other high-sodium foods in your diet. High blood pressure medicine is usually more effective when such a diet is properly followed.

Also, it may be very important for you to go on a reducing diet. However, check with your doctor before changing your diet.

• Many patients who have high blood pressure will not notice any signs of the problem. In fact, many may feel normal. It is very important that you **take your medicine exactly as directed** and that you keep your appointments with your doctor even if you feel well.

• Remember that this medicine will not cure your high blood pressure but it does help control it. Therefore, you must continue to take it as directed if you expect to lower your blood pressure and keep it down. **You may have to take high blood pressure medicine for the rest of your life.** If high blood pressure is not treated, it can cause serious problems such as heart failure, blood vessel disease, stroke, or kidney disease.

For patients taking the oral liquid form of hydrochlorothiazide, which comes in a dropper bottle:
• This medicine is to be taken by mouth. The amount you should take is to be measured only with the specially marked dropper.

If you miss a dose of this medicine, take it as soon as possible. However, if it is almost time for your next dose, skip the missed dose and go back to your regular dosing schedule. Do not double doses.

How to store this medicine:
• **Keep out of the reach of children.**
• Store away from heat and direct light.

• Do not store in the bathroom, near the kitchen sink, or in other damp places. Heat or moisture may cause the medicine to break down.

• Keep the oral liquid form of this medicine from freezing.

• Do not keep outdated medicine or medicine no longer needed. Be sure that any discarded medicine is out of the reach of children.

Precautions While Using This Medicine

It is important that your doctor check your progress at regular visits to make sure that this medicine is working properly.

This medicine may cause a loss of potassium from your body.

• To help prevent this, your doctor may want you to:

—eat or drink foods that have a high potassium content (for example, orange or other citrus fruit juices), or

—take a potassium supplement, or

—take another medicine to help prevent the loss of the potassium in the first place.

• It is very important to follow these directions. Also, it is important not to change your diet on your own. This is more important if you are already on a special diet (as for diabetes), or if you are taking a potassium supplement or a medicine to reduce potassium loss. Extra potassium may not be necessary and, in some cases, too much potassium could be harmful.

Check with your doctor if you become sick and have severe or continuing vomiting or diarrhea. These problems may cause you to lose additional water and potassium.

For diabetic patients:

• Thiazide diuretics may raise blood sugar levels. While you are using this medicine, be especially careful in testing for sugar in your blood or urine.

A few people who take this medicine may become more sensitive to sunlight than they are normally. When you first begin taking this medicine, avoid too much sun and do not use a sunlamp until you see how you react to the sun, especially if you tend to burn easily. If you have a severe reaction, check with your doctor.

For patients taking this medicine for high blood pressure:

• **Do not take other medicines unless they have been discussed with your doctor.** This especially includes over-the-counter (nonprescription) medicines for appetite control, asthma, colds, cough, hay fever, or sinus problems, since they may tend to increase your blood pressure.

Side Effects of This Medicine

Along with its needed effects, a medicine may cause some unwanted effects. Although not all of these side effects may occur, if they do occur they may need medical attention.

Check with your doctor as soon as possible if any of the following side effects occur:

Rare

Joint, lower back or side, or stomach pain
Skin rash or hives
Sore throat and fever
Stomach pain (severe) with nausea and vomiting
Unusual bleeding or bruising
Yellow eyes or skin

Signs and symptoms of too much potassium loss

Dryness of mouth
Increased thirst
Irregular heartbeats
Mood or mental changes
Muscle cramps or pain
Nausea or vomiting
Unusual tiredness or weakness
Weak pulse

Other side effects may occur that usually do not require medical attention. These side effects may go away during treatment as your body adjusts to the medicine. However, check with your doctor if any of the following side effects continue or are bothersome:

Less common

Decreased sexual ability

Diarrhea
Dizziness or lightheadedness when getting up from a lying
    or sitting position
Increased sensitivity of skin to sunlight
Loss of appetite
Upset stomach

For elderly patients:

• Some medicines may affect older patients differently than they do younger adults. Dizziness or lightheadedness and signs of too much potassium loss may
be more likely to occur in the elderly, who are more
sensitive to the effects of thiazide diuretics. Check
with your doctor if this occurs. In addition, it is a good
idea to check with your doctor or pharmacist if you
notice any unusual effects while you are taking this
medicine or if you think it is not working as it should.

Other side effects not listed above may also occur in some
patients. If you notice any other effects, check with
your doctor.

GUANABENZ (Systemic)†

A commonly used brand name in the U.S. is Wytensin.

†Not commercially available in Canada.

Guanabenz (GWAHN-a-benz) belongs to the general class of medicines called antihypertensives. It is taken by mouth to treat high blood pressure.

High blood pressure adds to the workload of the heart and arteries. If it continues for a long time, the heart and arteries may not function properly. This can damage the blood vessels of the brain, heart, and kidneys, resulting in a stroke, heart failure, or kidney failure. High blood pressure may also increase the risk of heart attacks. These problems may be less likely to occur if blood pressure is controlled.

Guanabenz works by controlling nerve impulses along certain nerve pathways. As a result, it relaxes blood vessels so that blood passes through them more easily. This helps to lower blood pressure.

Guanabenz is available only with your doctor's prescription.

Before Using This Medicine

To decide on the best treatment for your medical problem, your doctor should be told:

—if you have ever had any unusual or allergic reaction to guanabenz.

—if you are on a low-salt, low-sugar, or any other special diet, or if you are allergic to any substance, such as foods, sulfites or other preservatives, or dyes. Most medicines contain more than their active ingredient. Your doctor, nurse, or pharmacist can help you avoid products that may cause a problem.

—if you are **pregnant** or if you may become pregnant. Studies have not been done in humans. However, studies in rats have shown that guanabenz given in doses 9 to 10 times the maximum human dose caused a decrease in fertility. In addition, 3 to 6 times the maximum human dose caused birth defects (in the skeleton) in mice, and 6 to 9 times the maximum human dose caused death of the fetus in rats.

—if you are **breast-feeding**. It is not known whether guanabenz passes into the breast milk. However, this medicine has not been shown to cause problems in nursing babies.

—if you have any of the following medical problems:
Heart or blood vessel disease
Kidney disease
Liver disease

—if you are taking **any** other prescription or nonprescription (OTC) medicine, especially one that contains:
Beta-blockers (acebutolol [e.g., Sectral], atenolol [e.g., Tenormin], labetalol [e.g., Normodyne], metoprolol [e.g., Lopressor], nadolol [e.g., Corgard], oxprenolol [e.g., Trasicor], pindolol [e.g., Visken], propranolol [e.g., Inderal], sotalol [e.g., Sotacor], timolol [e.g., Blocadren])

Proper Use of This Medicine

Importance of diet—When prescribing medicine for your condition, your doctor may also prescribe a personal diet for you. Such a diet may be low in sodium (salt). Most people eat much more sodium than they need and too much sodium in the diet may increase blood pressure. Some foods that contain large amounts of sodium are canned soup, pickles, ketchup, green and ripe olives, relish, frankfurters, soy sauce, and carbonated beverages. Your doctor may want you to limit the amounts of these and other high-sodium foods in your diet. High blood pressure medicine is usually more effective when such a diet is properly followed.

Also, it may be very important for you to go on a reducing diet. However, check with your doctor before changing your diet.

Many patients who have high blood pressure will not notice any signs of the problem. In fact, many may feel normal. It is very important that you **take your medicine exactly as directed** and that you keep your appointments with your doctor even if you feel well.

Remember that this medicine will not cure your high blood pressure but it does help control it. Therefore, you must continue to take it as directed if you expect to lower your blood pressure and keep it down. **You may have to take high blood pressure medicine for the rest of your life.** If high blood pressure is not treated, it can cause serious problems such as heart failure, blood vessel disease, stroke, or kidney disease.

To help you remember to take your medicine, try to get into the habit of taking it at the same time each day.

If you miss a dose of this medicine, take it as soon as possible. However, if it is almost time for your next dose, skip the missed dose and go back to your regular dosing schedule. Do not double doses. If you miss two or more doses in a row, check with your doctor. If your body suddenly goes without this medicine, some unpleasant effects may occur. If you have any questions about this, check with your doctor.

How to store this medicine:

- **Keep out of the reach of children.**

- Store away from heat and direct light.

- Do not store in the bathroom, near the kitchen sink, or in other damp places. Heat or moisture may cause the medicine to break down.

- Do not keep outdated medicine or medicine no longer needed. Be sure that any discarded medicine is out of the reach of children.

Precautions While Using This Medicine

It is important that your doctor check your progress at regular visits to make sure that this medicine is working properly.

Check with your doctor before you stop taking guanabenz. Your doctor may want you to reduce gradually the amount you are taking before stopping completely.

Before having any kind of surgery (including dental surgery) or emergency treatment, tell the physician or dentist in charge that you are using this medicine.

Do not take other medicines unless they have been discussed with your doctor. This especially includes over-the-counter (nonprescription) medicines for appetite control, asthma, colds, cough, hay fever, or sinus problems, since they may tend to increase your blood pressure.

Guanabenz will add to the effects of alcohol and other CNS depressants (medicines that slow down the nervous system, possibly causing drowsiness). Some examples of CNS depressants are antihistamines or medicine for hay fever, other allergies, or colds; sedatives, tranquilizers, or sleeping medicine; prescription pain medicine or narcotics; barbiturates; medicine for seizures; muscle relaxants; or anesthetics, including some dental anesthetics. **Check with your doctor before taking any of the above while you are using this medicine.**

Guanabenz may cause some people to become dizzy, drowsy, or less alert than they are normally. **Make sure you know how you react to this medicine before you drive, use machines, or do other jobs that require you to be alert.**

Guanabenz may cause dryness of the mouth, nose, and throat. For temporary relief of mouth dryness, use sugarless candy or gum, melt bits of ice in your mouth, or use a saliva substitute. However, if dry mouth continues for more than 2 weeks, check with your physician or dentist. Continuing dryness of the mouth may increase the chance of dental disease, including tooth decay, gum disease, and fungus infections.

Side Effects of This Medicine

Along with its needed effects, a medicine may cause some unwanted effects. Although not all of these side effects may occur, if they do occur they may need medical attention.

Check with your doctor as soon as possible if any of the following side effects occur:

Signs and symptoms of overdose
   Dizziness (severe)
   Faintness
   Irritability
   Nervousness
   Pinpoint pupils

Slow heartbeat
Unusual tiredness or weakness

Other side effects may occur that usually do not require medical attention. These side effects may go away during treatment as your body adjusts to the medicine. However, check with your doctor if any of the following side effects continue or are bothersome:

More common

Dizziness
Drowsiness
Dry mouth
Weakness

Less common or rare

Decreased sexual ability
Headache
Nausea

After you have been using this medicine for a while, unpleasant effects may occur if you stop taking it too suddenly. After you stop taking this medicine, check with your doctor if any of the following effects occur:

Anxiety or tenseness
Chest pain
Fast or irregular heartbeat
Headache
Increased salivation
Increase in sweating
Nausea or vomiting
Nervousness or restlessness
Shaking or trembling of hands or fingers
Stomach cramps
Trouble in sleeping

For elderly patients:

• Some medicines may affect older patients differently than they do younger adults. Dizziness, faintness, or drowsiness may be more likely to occur in the elderly, who are usually more sensitive to the effects of guanabenz. Check with your doctor if this continues or is bothersome. In addition, it is a good idea to check with your doctor or pharmacist if you notice any unusual effects while taking this medicine or if you think it is not working as it should.

Other side effects not listed above may also occur in some patients. If you notice any other effects, check with your doctor.

GUANADREL (Systemic)†

A commonly used brand name in the U.S. is Hylorel.

---

†Not commercially available in Canada.

Guanadrel (GWAHN-a-drel) belongs to the general class of medicines called antihypertensives. It is used to treat high blood pressure.

High blood pressure adds to the workload of the heart and arteries. If it continues for a long time, the heart and arteries may not function properly. This can damage the blood vessels of the brain, heart, and kidneys resulting in a stroke, heart failure, or kidney failure. High blood pressure may also increase the risk of heart attacks. These problems may be less likely to occur if blood pressure is controlled.

Guanadrel works by controlling nerve impulses along certain nerve pathways. As a result, it relaxes the blood vessels so that blood passes through them more easily. This helps to lower blood pressure.

Guanadrel is available only with your doctor's prescription.

Before Using This Medicine

To decide on the best treatment for your medical problem, your doctor should be told:

—if you have ever had any unusual or allergic reaction to guanadrel.

—if you are on a low-salt, low-sugar, or any other special diet, or if you are allergic to any substance, such as foods, sulfites or other preservatives, or dyes. Most medicines contain more than their active ingredient. Your doctor, nurse, or pharmacist can help you avoid products that may cause a problem.

—if you are **pregnant** or if you may become pregnant. Studies have not been done in humans. However, guanadrel has not been shown to cause birth defects or other problems in rats and rabbits given up to 12 times the highest human dose.

—if you are **breast-feeding**. It is not known whether guanadrel passes into breast milk. However, it has not been shown to cause problems in nursing babies.

—if you have any of the following medical problems:
   Asthma (history of)
   Diarrhea
   Fever
   Heart or blood vessel disease
   Pheochromocytoma
   Stomach ulcer (history of)

—if you have recently had a heart attack or stroke.

—if you are taking **any** other prescription or nonprescription (OTC) medicine, especially one that contains:
   Chlorprothixene (e.g., Taractan)
   Loxapine (e.g., Loxitane)
   Thiothixene (e.g., Navane)
   Tricyclic antidepressants (amitriptyline [e.g., Elavil], amox-
       apine [e.g., Asendin], clomipramine [e.g., Anafranil], de-
       sipramine [e.g., Pertofrane], doxepin [e.g., Sinequan],
       imipramine [e.g., Tofranil], nortriptyline [e.g., Aventyl],
       protriptyline [e.g., Vivactil], trimipramine [e.g., Surmon-
       til])
   Trimeprazine (e.g., Temaril)

—if you are now taking or have taken within the past **2** weeks monoamine oxidase (MAO) inhibitors such as:
   Furazolidone (e.g., Furoxone)
   Isocarboxazid (e.g., Marplan)
   Pargyline (e.g., Eutonyl)
   Phenelzine (e.g., Nardil)
   Procarbazine (e.g., Matulane)
   Tranylcypromine (e.g., Parnate)

Proper Use of This Medicine

Importance of diet—When prescribing medicine for your condition, your doctor may also prescribe a personal diet for you. Such a diet may be low in sodium (salt). Most people eat much more sodium than they need and too much sodium in the diet may increase blood pressure. Some foods that contain large amounts of sodium are canned soup, pickles, ketchup, green and ripe olives, rel-ish, frankfurters, soy sauce, and carbonated beverages. Your doctor may want you to limit the amounts of these and other high-sodium foods in your diet. High blood pressure medicine is usually more effective when such a diet is properly followed.

Also, it may be very important for you to go on a reducing diet. However, check with your doctor before changing your diet.

Many patients who have high blood pressure will not notice any signs of the problem. In fact, many may feel normal. It is very important that you **take your medicine exactly as directed** and that you keep your appointments with your doctor even if you feel well.

Remember that guanadrel will not cure your high blood pressure but it does help control it. Therefore, you must continue to take it as directed if you expect to lower your blood pressure and keep it down. **You may have to take high blood pressure medicine for the rest of your life.** If high blood pressure is not treated, it can cause serious problems such as heart failure, blood vessel disease, stroke, or kidney disease.

To help you remember to take your medicine, try to get into the habit of taking it at the same time each day.

If you miss a dose of guanadrel, take it as soon as possible. However, if it is almost time for your next dose, skip the missed dose and go back to your regular dosing schedule. Do not double doses.

How to store this medicine:
• **Keep out of the reach of children.**

• Store away from heat and direct light.

• Do not store in the bathroom, near the kitchen sink, or in other damp places. Heat or moisture may cause the medicine to break down.

• Do not keep outdated medicine or medicine no longer needed. Be sure that any discarded medicine is out of the reach of children.

Precautions While Using This Medicine

It is important that your doctor check your progress at regular visits to make sure that this medicine is working properly.

Dizziness, lightheadedness, or fainting may occur, especially when you get up from a lying or sitting position. This may be more likely to occur in the morning. **Getting up slowly may help.** If you feel dizzy, sit or lie down. When you get up from lying down, sit on the edge of the bed with your feet dangling for 1 or 2 minutes. Then stand up slowly. If the problem continues or gets worse, check with your doctor.

The dizziness, lightheadedness, or fainting is also more likely to occur if you drink alcohol, stand for long periods of time, exercise, or if the weather is hot. **While you are taking guanadrel, be careful in the amount of alcohol you drink. Also, use extra care during exercise or hot weather or if you must stand for long periods of time.**

Do not take other medicines unless they have been discussed with your doctor. This especially includes over-the-counter (nonprescription) medicines for appetite control, asthma, colds, cough, hay fever, or sinus problems, since they may tend to increase your blood pressure.

Before having any kind of surgery (including dental surgery) or emergency treatment, tell the physician or dentist in charge that you are taking guanadrel.

Tell your doctor if you get a fever since that may change the amount of medicine you have to take.

Side Effects of This Medicine

Along with its needed effects, a medicine may cause some unwanted effects. Although not all of these side effects may occur, if they do occur they may need medical attention.

Check with your doctor immediately if either of the following side effects occurs since they may be symptoms of an overdose:

Rare

　　Blurred vision
　　Dizziness or faintness (severe)

Check with your doctor as soon as possible if any of the following side effects occur:

More common
Swelling of feet or lower legs

Less common or rare
Chest pain
Shortness of breath

Other side effects may occur that usually do not require medical attention. These side effects may go away during treatment as your body adjusts to the medicine. However, check with your doctor if any of the following side effects continue or are bothersome:

More common
Difficulty in ejaculating
Dizziness, lightheadedness, or fainting, especially when getting up from a lying or sitting position
Drowsiness or tiredness

Less common or rare
Diarrhea or increase in bowel movements
Dry mouth
Headache
Muscle pain or tremors
Nighttime urination

For elderly patients:
• Some medicines may affect older patients differently than they do younger adults. Dizziness or faintness may be more likely to occur in the elderly, who are usually more sensitive to the effects of guanadrel. Check with your doctor if this continues or is bothersome. In addition, it is a good idea to check with your doctor or pharmacist if you notice any unusual effects while taking this medicine or if you think it is not working as it should.

Other side effects not listed above may also occur in some patients. If you notice any other effects, check with your doctor.

GUANETHIDINE (Systemic)

Some commonly used brand names are:

In the U.S.
    Ismelin
    Generic name product may also be available.

In Canada
    Apo-Guanethidine
    Ismelin

Guanethidine (gwahn-ETH-i-deen) belongs to the general class of medicines called antihypertensives. It is taken by mouth to treat high blood pressure. High blood pressure adds to the workload of the heart and arteries. If it continues for a long time, the heart and arteries may not function properly. This can damage the blood vessels of the brain, heart, and kidneys, resulting in a stroke, heart failure, or kidney failure. High blood pressure may also increase the risk of heart attacks. These problems may be less likely to occur if blood pressure is controlled.

Guanethidine works by controlling nerve impulses along certain nerve pathways. As a result, it relaxes the blood vessels so that blood passes through them more easily. This helps to lower blood pressure.

Guanethidine is available only with your doctor's prescription.

Before Using This Medicine

To decide on the best treatment for your medical problem, your doctor should be told:

—if you have ever had any unusual or allergic reaction to guanethidine.

—if you are on a low-salt, low-sugar, or any other special diet, or if you are allergic to any substance, such as foods, sulfites or other preservatives, or dyes. Most medicines contain more than their active ingredient. Your doctor, nurse, or pharmacist can help you avoid products that may cause a problem.

—if you are **pregnant** or if you may become pregnant. Studies have not been done in either humans or animals.

—if you are **breast-feeding**. Guanethidine has not been shown to cause problems in nursing babies.

—if you have any of the following medical problems:
 Asthma (history of)
 Diabetes mellitus (sugar diabetes)
 Diarrhea
 Fever
 Heart or blood vessel disease
 Kidney disease
 Liver disease
 Pheochromocytoma
 Stomach ulcer (history of)

—if you have recently had a heart attack or stroke.

—if you are now taking or have taken within the past 2 weeks monoamine oxidase (MAO) inhibitors such as:
 Furazolidone (e.g., Furoxone)
 Isocarboxazid (e.g., Marplan)
 Pargyline (e.g., Eutonyl)
 Phenelzine (e.g., Nardil)
 Procarbazine (e.g., Matulane)
 Tranylcypromine (e.g., Parnate)

—if you are taking **any** other prescription or nonprescription (OTC) medicine, especially one that contains:
 Antidiabetics, oral (diabetes medicine you take by mouth)
 Chlorprothixene (e.g., Taractan)
 Loxapine (e.g., Loxitane)
 Minoxidil (e.g., Loniten)
 Thiothixene (e.g., Navane)
 Tricyclic antidepressants (amitriptyline [e.g., Elavil], amoxapine [e.g., Asendin], clomipramine [e.g., Anafranil], desipramine [e.g., Pertofrane], doxepin [e.g., Sinequan], imipramine [e.g., Tofranil], nortriptyline [e.g., Aventyl], protriptyline [e.g., Vivactil], trimipramine [e.g., Surmontil])

Proper Use of This Medicine

Importance of diet—When prescribing medicine for your condition, your doctor may also prescribe a personal diet for you. Such a diet may be low in sodium (salt). Most people eat much more sodium than they need and too much sodium in the diet may increase blood pressure. Some foods that contain large amounts of sodium are canned soup, pickles, ketchup, green and ripe olives, relish, frankfurters, soy sauce, and carbonated beverages.

Your doctor may want you to limit the amounts of these and other high-sodium foods in your diet. High blood pressure medicine is usually more effective when such a diet is properly followed.

Also, it may be very important for you to go on a reducing diet. However, check with your doctor before changing your diet.

Many patients who have high blood pressure will not notice any signs of the problem. In fact, many may feel normal. It is very important that you **take your medicine exactly as directed** and that you keep your appointments with your doctor even if you feel well.

Remember that guanethidine will not cure your high blood pressure but it does help control it. Therefore, you must continue to take it as directed if you expect to lower your blood pressure and keep it down. **You may have to take high blood pressure medicine for the rest of your life.** If high blood pressure is not treated, it can cause serious problems such as heart failure, blood vessel disease, stroke, or kidney disease.

To help you remember to take your medicine, try to get into the habit of taking it at the same time each day.

If you miss a dose of guanethidine, take it as soon as possible. However, if it is almost time for your next dose, skip the missed dose and go back to your regular dosing schedule. Do not double doses.

How to store this medicine:

- **Keep out of the reach of children.**

- Store away from heat and direct light.

- Do not store in the bathroom, near the kitchen sink, or in other damp places. Heat or moisture may cause the medicine to break down.

- Do not keep outdated medicine or medicine no longer needed. Be sure that any discarded medicine is out of the reach of children.

Precautions While Using This Medicine

It is important that your doctor check your progress at regular visits to make sure that this medicine is working properly.

Dizziness, lightheadedness, or fainting may occur, especially when you get up from a lying or sitting position. This is more likely to occur in the morning. **Getting up slowly may help.** When you get up from lying down, sit on the edge of the bed with your feet dangling for 1 or 2 minutes. Then stand up slowly. If the problem continues or gets worse, check with your doctor.

The dizziness, lightheadedness, or fainting is also more likely to occur if you drink alcohol, stand for long periods of time, exercise, or if the weather is hot. **While you are taking this medicine, be careful in the amount of alcohol you drink. Also, use extra care during exercise or hot weather or if you must stand for long periods of time.**

Do not take other medicines unless they have been discussed with your doctor. This especially includes over-the-counter (nonprescription) medicines for appetite control, asthma, colds, cough, hay fever, or sinus problems, since they may tend to increase your blood pressure.

Before having any kind of surgery (including dental surgery) or emergency treatment, tell the physician or dentist in charge that you are taking this medicine.

Tell your doctor if you get a fever since that may change the amount of medicine you have to take.

Side Effects of This Medicine

Along with its needed effects, a medicine may cause some unwanted effects. Although not all of these side effects may occur, if they do occur they may need medical attention.

Check with your doctor as soon as possible if any of the following side effects occur:
More common
    Swelling of feet or lower legs

Less common or rare
Chest pain
Shortness of breath

Other side effects may occur that usually do not require medical attention. These side effects may go away during treatment as your body adjusts to the medicine. However, check with your doctor if any of the following side effects continue or are bothersome:

More common
Diarrhea or increase in bowel movements
Dizziness, lightheadedness, or fainting, especially when getting up from a lying or sitting position
Sexual problems in males
Slow heartbeat
Stuffy nose
Unusual tiredness or weakness

Less common or rare
Blurred vision
Drooping eyelids
Dry mouth
Headache
Loss of hair on scalp
Muscle pain or tremors
Nausea or vomiting
Nighttime urination
Skin rash

For elderly patients:

• Some medicines may affect older patients differently than they do younger adults. Dizziness, lightheadedness, or fainting may be more likely to occur in the elderly, who are more sensitive to the effects of guanethidine. Check with your doctor if this continues or is bothersome. In addition, it is a good idea to check with your doctor or pharmacist if you notice any unusual effects while taking this medicine or if you think it is not working as it should.

Other side effects not listed above may also occur in some patients. If you notice any other effects, check with your doctor.

GUANETHIDINE AND
HYDROCHLOROTHIAZIDE (Systemic)

A commonly used brand name in the U.S. is Esimil.

Guanethidine (gwahn-ETH-i-deen) and hydrochlorothiazide (hye-droe-klor-oh-THYE-a-zide) combination is taken by mouth to treat high blood pressure.

High blood pressure adds to the workload of the heart and arteries. If it continues for a long time, the heart and arteries may not function properly. This can damage the blood vessels of the brain, heart, and kidneys, resulting in a stroke, heart failure, or kidney failure. High blood pressure may also increase the risk of heart attacks. These problems may be less likely to occur if blood pressure is controlled.

Guanethidine works by controlling nerve impulses along certain nerve pathways. As a result, it relaxes the blood vessels so that blood passes through them more easily. The hydrochlorothiazide in this combination is a thiazide diuretic (water pill) that helps reduce the amount of water in the body by increasing the flow of urine.

Guanethidine and hydrochlorothiazide combination is available only with your doctor's prescription.

Before Using This Medicine

To decide on the best treatment for your medical problem, your doctor should be told:

—if you have ever had any unusual or allergic reaction to guanethidine, sulfonamides (sulfa drugs), hydrochlorothiazide, or other thiazide diuretics (water pills).

—if you are on a low-salt, low-sugar, or any other special diet, or if you are allergic to any substance, such as foods, sulfites or other preservatives, or dyes. Most medicines contain more than their active ingredient. Your doctor, nurse, or pharmacist can help you avoid products that may cause a problem.

—if you are **pregnant** or if you may become pregnant. When hydrochlorothiazide is used during pregnancy, it may cause side effects including jaundice, blood problems, and low potassium in the newborn infant. However, this medicine has not been shown to cause birth defects.

—if you are **breast-feeding**. Although hydrochlorothiazide passes into breast milk, this medicine has not been shown to cause problems in nursing babies.

—if you have any of the following medical problems:
Asthma (history of)
Diabetes mellitus (sugar diabetes)
Diarrhea
Fever
Gout
Heart or blood vessel disease
Kidney disease
Liver disease
Lupus erythematosus (history of)
Pancreatitis (inflammation of the pancreas)
Pheochromocytoma
Stomach ulcer (history of)

—if you have recently had a heart attack or stroke.

—if you are now taking or have taken within the past 2 weeks monoamine oxidase (MAO) inhibitors such as:
Furazolidone (e.g., Furoxone)
Isocarboxazid (e.g., Marplan)
Pargyline (e.g., Eutonyl)
Phenelzine (e.g., Nardil)
Procarbazine (e.g., Matulane)
Tranylcypromine (e.g., Parnate)

—if you are taking **any** other prescription or nonprescription (OTC) medicine, especially one that contains:
Adrenocorticoids (cortisone-like medicines)
Antidiabetics, oral (diabetes medicine you take by mouth)
Chlorprothixene (e.g., Taractan)
Lithium (e.g., Lithane)
Loxapine (e.g., Loxitane)
Methenamine (e.g., Mandelamine)
Thiothixene (e.g., Navane)
Tricyclic antidepressants (amitriptyline [e.g., Elavil], amoxapine [e.g., Asendin], clomipramine [e.g., Anafranil], desipramine [e.g., Pertofrane], doxepin [e.g., Sinequan], imipramine [e.g., Tofranil], nortriptyline [e.g., Aventyl], protriptyline [e.g., Vivactil], trimipramine [e.g., Surmontil])

Proper Use of This Medicine

This medicine may cause you to have an unusual feeling of tiredness when you begin to take it. You may also notice an increase in the amount of urine or in your frequency of urination. After taking the medicine for a while, these effects should lessen. In general, in order to keep the increase in urine from affecting your sleep:

• If you are to take a single dose a day, take it in the morning after breakfast.

• If you are to take more than one dose a day, take the last dose no later than 6 p.m., unless otherwise directed by your doctor.

However, it is best to plan your dose or doses according to a schedule that will least affect your personal activities and sleep. Ask your doctor, nurse, or pharmacist to help you plan the best time to take this medicine.

Importance of diet—When prescribing medicine for your condition, your doctor may also prescribe a personal diet for you. Such a diet may be low in sodium (salt). Most people eat much more sodium than they need and too much sodium in the diet may increase blood pressure. Some foods that contain large amounts of sodium are canned soup, pickles, ketchup, green and ripe olives, relish, frankfurters, soy sauce, and carbonated beverages. Your doctor may want you to limit the amounts of these and other high-sodium foods in your diet. High blood pressure medicine is usually more effective when such a diet is properly followed.

Also, it may be very important for you to go on a reducing diet. However, check with your doctor before changing your diet.

Many patients who have high blood pressure will not notice any signs of the problem. In fact, many may feel normal. It is very important that you **take your medicine exactly as directed** and that you keep your appointments with your doctor even if you feel well.

Remember that this medicine will not cure your high blood pressure but it does help control it. Therefore, you must continue to take it as directed if you expect to lower your blood pressure and keep it down. **You may have to take high blood pressure medicine for the rest of your life.** If high blood pressure is not treated, it can cause serious

problems such as heart failure, blood vessel disease, stroke, or kidney disease.

To help you remember to take your medicine, try to get into the habit of taking it at the same time each day.

If you miss a dose of this medicine, take it as soon as possible. However, if it is almost time for your next dose, skip the missed dose and go back to your regular dosing schedule. Do not double doses.

How to store this medicine:

- **Keep out of the reach of children.**

- Store away from heat and direct light.

- Do not store in the bathroom, near the kitchen sink, or in other damp places. Heat or moisture may cause the medicine to break down.

- Do not keep outdated medicine or medicine no longer needed. Be sure that any discarded medicine is out of the reach of children.

Precautions While Using This Medicine

It is important that your doctor check your progress at regular visits to make sure that this medicine is working properly.

Do not take other medicines unless they have been discussed with your doctor. This especially includes over-the-counter (nonprescription) medicines for appetite control, asthma, colds, cough, hay fever, or sinus problems, since they may tend to increase your blood pressure.

This medicine may cause a loss of potassium from your body.

- To help prevent this, your doctor may want you to:

    —eat or drink foods that have a high potassium content (for example, orange or other citrus fruit juices), or

    —take a potassium supplement, or

    —take another medicine to help prevent the loss of the potassium in the first place.

• It is very important to follow these directions. Also, it is important not to change your diet on your own. This is more important if you are already on a special diet (as for diabetes), or if you are taking a potassium supplement or a medicine to reduce potassium loss. Extra potassium may not be necessary and, in some cases, too much potassium could be harmful.

Check with your doctor if you become sick and have severe or continuing vomiting or diarrhea. These problems may cause you to lose additional water and potassium.

Dizziness, lightheadedness, or fainting may occur, especially when you get up from a lying or sitting position. This is more likely to occur in the morning. **Getting up slowly** may help. When you get up from lying down, sit on the edge of the bed with your feet dangling for 1 or 2 minutes. Then stand up slowly. If the problem continues or gets worse, check with your doctor.

The dizziness, lightheadedness, or fainting is also more likely to occur if you drink alcohol, stand for long periods of time or exercise, or if the weather is hot. **While you are taking this medicine, be careful in the amount of alcohol you drink. Also, use extra care during exercise or hot weather or if you must stand for long periods of time.**

For diabetic patients:
• This medicine may raise blood sugar levels. While you are using this medicine, be especially careful in testing for sugar in your blood or urine. If you have any questions about this, check with your doctor.

Some people who take this medicine may become more sensitive to sunlight than they are normally. When you first begin taking this medicine, avoid too much sun and do not use a sunlamp until you see how you react to the sun, especially if you tend to burn easily. If you have a severe reaction, check with your doctor.

Tell your doctor if you get a fever since that may change the amount of medicine you have to take.

Before having any kind of surgery (including dental surgery) or emergency treatment, tell the physician or dentist in charge that you are taking this medicine.

Side Effects of This Medicine

Along with its needed effects, a medicine may cause some unwanted effects. Although not all of these side effects may occur, if they do occur they may need medical attention.

Check with your doctor as soon as possible if any of the following side effects occur, especially since some of them may mean that your body is losing too much potassium:

Signs and symptoms of too much potassium loss
>Dryness of mouth
>Increased thirst
>Irregular heartbeats
>Mood or mental changes
>Muscle cramps or pain
>Nausea or vomiting
>Unusual tiredness or weakness
>Weak pulse

Less common
>Chest pain

Rare
>Joint, lower back or side, or stomach pain
>Skin rash or hives
>Sore throat and fever
>Stomach pain (severe) with nausea and vomiting
>Unusual bleeding or bruising
>Yellow eyes or skin

Other side effects may occur that usually do not require medical attention. These side effects may go away during treatment as your body adjusts to the medicine. However, check with your doctor if any of the following side effects continue or are bothersome:

More common
>Diarrhea or increase in bowel movements
>Dizziness, lightheadedness, or fainting, especially when getting up from a lying or sitting position
>Sexual problems in males

Slow heartbeat
Stuffy nose

Less common or rare

Blurred vision
Drooping eyelids
Headache
Increased sensitivity to sunlight
Loss of appetite
Loss of hair
Nighttime urination

For elderly patients:

• Some medicines may affect older patients differently than they do younger adults. Dizziness, lightheadedness, fainting, or signs and symptoms of too much potassium loss may be more likely to occur in the elderly, who are more sensitive to the effects of guanethidine and hydrochlorothiazide. Check with your doctor if these continue or are bothersome. In addition, it is a good idea to check with your doctor or pharmacist if you notice any unusual effects while taking this medicine or if you think it is not working as it should.

Other side effects not listed above may also occur in some patients. If you notice any other effects, check with your doctor.

GUANFACINE (Systemic)†

A commonly used brand name in the U.S. is Tenex.

---

†Not commercially available in Canada.

Guanfacine (GWAHN-fa-seen) belongs to the general class of medicines called antihypertensives. It is used to treat high blood pressure. High blood pressure adds to the workload of the heart and arteries. If it continues for a long time, the heart and arteries may not function properly. This can damage the blood vessels of the brain, heart, and kidneys, resulting in a stroke, heart failure, or kidney failure. High blood pressure may also increase the risk of heart attacks. These problems may be less likely to occur if blood pressure is controlled.

Guanfacine works by controlling nerve impulses along certain nerve pathways. As a result, it relaxes blood vessels so that blood passes through them more easily. This helps to lower blood pressure.

Guanfacine is available only with your doctor's prescription.

Before Using This Medicine

To decide on the best treatment for your medical problem, your doctor should be told:

—if you have ever had any unusual or allergic reaction to guanfacine.

—if you are on a low-salt, low-sugar, or any other special diet, or if you are allergic to any substance, such as foods, sulfites or other preservatives, or dyes. Most medicines contain more than their active ingredient. Your doctor, nurse, or pharmacist can help you avoid products that may cause a problem.

—if you are **pregnant** or if you may become pregnant. Studies have not been done in humans. However, guanfacine has not been shown to cause birth defects or other problems in rats or rabbits given many times the human dose. In rats and rabbits given extremely high doses (up to 200 times the human dose), there was an increase in deaths of the animal fetus.

—if you are **breast-feeding**. It is not known whether guan-facine passes into the breast milk. It has not been shown to cause problems in nursing babies.

—if you have any of the following medical problems:
   Heart disease
   Liver disease
   Mental depression

—if you have recently had a heart attack or stroke.

—if you are taking **any** other prescription or nonprescription (OTC) medicine.

Proper Use of This Medicine

Importance of diet—When prescribing medicine for your condition, your doctor may also prescribe a personal diet for you. Such a diet may be low in sodium (salt). Most people eat much more sodium than they need and too much sodium in the diet may increase blood pressure. Some foods that contain large amounts of sodium are canned soup, pickles, ketchup, green and ripe olives, rel-ish, frankfurters, soy sauce, and carbonated beverages. Your doctor may want you to limit the amounts of these and other high-sodium foods in your diet. High blood pressure medicine is usually more effective when such a diet is properly followed.

Also, it may be very important for you to go on a reducing diet. However, check with your doctor before changing your diet.

Many patients who have high blood pressure will not notice any signs of the problem. In fact, many may feel normal. It is very important that you **take your medicine exactly as directed** and that you keep your appointments with your doctor even if you feel well.

Remember that this medicine will not cure your high blood pressure but it does help control it. Therefore, you must continue to use it as directed if you expect to lower your blood pressure and keep it down. **You may have to take high blood pressure medicine for the rest of your life.** If high blood pressure is not treated, it can cause serious

problems such as heart failure, blood vessel disease, stroke, or kidney disease.

Take your daily dose of guanfacine at bedtime. (If you are taking more than one dose a day, take your last dose at bedtime). Taking it this way will help lessen daytime drowsiness.

If you miss a dose of this medicine, take it as soon as possible. However, if it is almost time for your next dose, skip the missed dose and go back to your regular dosing schedule. Do not double doses. **If you miss taking guanfacine for two or more days in a row, check with your doctor.** If your body suddenly goes without this medicine, some unwanted effects may occur. If you have any questions about this, check with your doctor.

How to store this medicine:

• **Keep out of the reach of children.**

• Store away from heat and direct light.

• Do not store in the bathroom, near the kitchen sink, or in other damp places. Heat or moisture may cause the medicine to break down.

• Do not keep outdated medicine or medicine no longer needed. Be sure any discarded medicine is out of the reach of children.

Precautions While Using This Medicine

It is important that your doctor check your progress at regular visits to make sure this medicine is working properly.

Check with your doctor before you stop taking guanfacine. Your doctor may want you to reduce gradually the amount you are taking before stopping completely.

Make sure that you have enough guanfacine on hand to last through weekends, holidays, and vacations. You should not miss any doses. You may want to ask your doctor for another written prescription for guanfacine to carry in your wallet or purse. You can then have it filled if you run out when you are away from home.

Before having any kind of surgery (including dental surgery) or emergency treatment, tell the physician or dentist in charge that you are using this medicine.

Do not take other medicines unless they have been discussed with your doctor. This especially includes over-the-counter (nonprescription) medicines for appetite control, asthma, colds, cough, hay fever, or sinus problems, since they may tend to increase your blood pressure.

Guanfacine will add to the effects of alcohol and other CNS depressants (medicines that slow down the nervous system, possibly causing drowsiness). Some examples of CNS depressants are antihistamines or medicine for hay fever, other allergies, or colds; sedatives, tranquilizers, or sleeping medicine; prescription pain medicine or narcotics; barbiturates; medicine for seizures; muscle relaxants; or anesthetics, including some dental anesthetics. **Check with your doctor before taking any of the above while you are using this medicine.**

Guanfacine may cause some people to become dizzy, drowsy, or less alert than they are normally. **Make sure you know how you react to this medicine before you drive, use machines, or do other jobs that could be dangerous if you are not alert.**

Guanfacine may cause dryness of the mouth, nose, and throat. For temporary relief of mouth dryness, use sugarless candy or gum, melt bits of ice in your mouth, or use a saliva substitute. However, if dry mouth continues for more than 2 weeks, check with your physician or dentist. Continuing dryness of the mouth may increase the chance of dental disease, including tooth decay, gum disease, and fungus infections.

Side Effects of This Medicine

Along with its needed effects, a medicine may cause some unwanted effects. Although not all of these side effects may occur, if they do occur they may need medical attention.

Check with your doctor as soon as possible if any of the following side effects occur:

Less common
- Confusion
- Mental depression

Signs and symptoms of overdose
- Difficulty in breathing
- Dizziness (extreme) or faintness
- Slow heartbeat
- Unusual tiredness or weakness (severe)

Other side effects may occur that usually do not require medical attention. These side effects may go away during treatment as your body adjusts to the medicine. However, check with your doctor if any of the following side effects continue or are bothersome:

More common
- Constipation
- Dizziness
- Drowsiness
- Dry mouth

Less common
- Decreased sexual ability
- Dry, itching, or burning eyes
- Headache
- Nausea or vomiting
- Trouble in sleeping
- Unusual tiredness or weakness

After you have been using this medicine for a while, unwanted effects may occur if you stop taking it too suddenly. After you stop taking this medicine, check with your doctor if any of the following side effects occur:
- Anxiety or tenseness
- Chest pain
- Fast or irregular heartbeat
- Headache
- Increased salivation
- Nausea or vomiting
- Nervousness or restlessness
- Shaking or trembling of hands and fingers

Stomach cramps
Sweating
Trouble in sleeping

For elderly patients:

• Some medicines may affect older patients differently than they do younger adults. Dizziness, drowsiness, or faintness may be more likely to occur in the elderly, who are more sensitive to the effects of guanfacine. Check with your doctor if this continues or is bothersome. In addition, it is a good idea to check with your doctor or pharmacist if you notice any unusual effects while taking this medicine or if you think it is not working as it should.

Other side effects not listed above may also occur in some patients. If you notice any other effects, check with your doctor.

HYDRALAZINE (Systemic)

Some commonly used brand names are:

In the U.S.
>   Apresoline
> Generic name product may also be available.

In Canada
>   Apresoline
>   Novo-Hylazin

Hydralazine (hye-DRAL-a-zeen) belongs to the general class of medicines called antihypertensives. It is used to treat high blood pressure.

High blood pressure adds to the workload of the heart and arteries. If it continues for a long time, the heart and arteries may not function properly. This can damage the blood vessels of the brain, heart, and kidneys, resulting in a stroke, heart failure, or kidney failure. High blood pressure may also increase the risk of heart attacks. These problems may be less likely to occur if blood pressure is controlled.

Hydralazine works by relaxing blood vessels and increasing the supply of blood and oxygen to the heart while reducing its work load.

Hydralazine may also be used for other conditions as determined by your doctor.

Hydralazine is available only with your doctor's prescription.

Before Using This Medicine

To decide on the best treatment for your medical problem, your doctor should be told:

—if you have ever had any unusual or allergic reaction to hydralazine.

—if you are on a low-salt, low-sugar, or any other special diet, or if you are allergic to any substance, such as foods, sulfites or other preservatives, or dyes. Most medicines contain more than their active ingredient. Your doctor, nurse, or pharmacist can help you avoid products that may cause a problem.

—if you are **pregnant** or if you may become pregnant. Studies have not been done in humans. However, studies in mice have shown that hydralazine causes birth defects (cleft palate, defects in head and face bones). These birth defects may also occur in rabbits, but do not occur in rats.

—if you are **breast-feeding**. Hydralazine has not been shown to cause problems in nursing babies.

—if you have either of the following medical problems:
Heart or blood vessel disease
Kidney disease

—if you have recently had a stroke.

—if you are taking **any** other prescription or nonprescription (OTC) medicine, especially diazoxide (e.g., Proglycem).

Proper Use of This Medicine

For patients taking this medicine for high blood pressure:

• Importance of diet—When prescribing medicine for your condition, your doctor may also prescribe a personal diet for you. Such a diet may be low in sodium (salt). Most people eat much more sodium than they need and too much sodium in the diet may increase blood pressure. Some foods that contain large amounts of sodium are canned soup, pickles, ketchup, green and ripe olives, relish, frankfurters, soy sauce, and carbonated beverages. Your doctor may want you to limit the amounts of these and other high-sodium foods in your diet. High blood pressure medicine is usually more effective when such a diet is properly followed.

Also, it may be very important for you to go on a reducing diet. However, check with your doctor before changing your diet.

• Many patients who have high blood pressure will not notice any signs of the problem. In fact, many may feel normal. It is very important that you **take your medicine exactly as directed** and that you keep your appointments with your doctor even if you feel well.

• Remember that hydralazine will not cure your high blood pressure but it does help control it. Therefore, you must continue to take it as directed if you expect to lower your blood pressure and keep it down. **You may have to**

take high blood pressure medicine for the rest of your life.
If high blood pressure is not treated, it can cause serious
problems such as heart failure, blood vessel disease, stroke,
or kidney disease.

To help you remember to take your medicine, try to get into
the habit of taking it at the same time each day.

If you miss a dose of this medicine, take it as soon as possible.
However, if it is almost time for your next dose, skip the
missed dose and go back to your regular dosing schedule.
Do not double doses.

How to store this medicine:

• **Keep out of the reach of children.**

• Store away from heat and direct light.

• Do not store in the bathroom, near the kitchen sink, or
in other damp places. Heat or moisture may cause the
medicine to break down.

• Do not keep outdated medicine or medicine no longer
needed. Be sure that any discarded medicine is out of the
reach of children.

Precautions While Using This Medicine

It is important that your doctor check your progress at regular visits to make sure that this medicine is working
properly.

For patients taking this medicine for high blood pressure:
• **Do not take other medicines unless they have been discussed with your doctor.** This especially includes over-
the-counter (nonprescription) medicines for appetite control, asthma, colds, cough, hay fever, or sinus, since they
may tend to increase your blood pressure.

Hydralazine may cause some people to have headaches or
to feel dizzy. **Make sure you know how you react to this
medicine before you drive, use machines, or do other jobs
that could be dangerous if you are not alert.**

Side Effects of This Medicine

Along with its needed effects, a medicine may cause some unwanted effects. Although not all of these side effects may occur, if they do occur they may need medical attention.

In general, side effects with hydralazine are rare at lower doses. However, check with your doctor as soon as possible if any of the following occur:

Less common

    Blisters on skin
    Chest pain
    General feeling of body discomfort or weakness
    Joint pain
    Numbness, tingling, pain, or weakness in hands or feet
    Skin rash or itching
    Sore throat and fever
    Swelling of feet or lower legs
    Swelling of the lymph glands

Other side effects may occur that usually do not require medical attention. These side effects may go away during treatment as your body adjusts to the medicine. However, check with your doctor if any of the following side effects continue or are bothersome:

More common

    Diarrhea
    Fast or irregular heartbeat
    Headache
    Loss of appetite
    Nausea or vomiting

Less common

    Constipation
    Dizziness or lightheadedness
    Redness or flushing of face
    Shortness of breath with exercise or work
    Stuffy nose
    Watering or irritated eyes

For elderly patients:

    • Some medicines may affect older patients differently than they do younger adults. Dizziness or lightheadedness may be more likely to occur in the elderly, who are more sensitive to the effects of hydralazine. Check with your doctor if this continues or is bothersome. Also, hydralazine may reduce tolerance to cold temperatures in elderly patients. Check with your doctor if this occurs. In addition, it is a good idea to check with your doctor or pharmacist if you notice any other unusual effects while taking this medicine or if you think it is not working as it should.

Other side effects not listed above may also occur in some patients. If you notice any other effects, check with your doctor.

HYDRALAZINE AND HYDROCHLOROTHIAZIDE
(Systemic)

Some commonly used brand names in the U.S. are:

Apresazide	Aprozide
Apresodex	Hydra-zide
Apresoline-Esidrix	

Generic name product may also be available in the U.S.

Hydralazine (hye-DRAL-a-zeen) and hydrochlorothiazide (hye-droe-klor-oh-THYE-a-zide) combination is taken by mouth to treat high blood pressure.

High blood pressure adds to the workload of the heart and arteries. If it continues for a long time, the heart and arteries may not function properly. This can damage the blood vessels of the brain, heart, and kidneys, resulting in a stroke, heart failure, or kidney failure. High blood pressure may also increase the risk of heart attacks. These problems may be less likely to occur if blood pressure is controlled.

Hydralazine works by relaxing blood vessels and increasing the supply of blood and oxygen to the heart while reducing its work load. The hydrochlorothiazide in this combination helps reduce the amount of water in the body by acting on the kidneys to increase the flow of urine.

This medicine is available only with your doctor's prescription.

Before Using This Medicine

To decide on the best treatment for your medical problem, your doctor should be told:

—if you have ever had any unusual or allergic reaction to hydralazine, sulfonamides (sulfa drugs), indapamide, or any of the thiazide diuretics (water pills).

—if you are on a low-salt, low-sugar, or any other special diet, or if you are allergic to any substance, such as foods, sulfites or other preservatives, or dyes. Most medicines contain more than their active ingredient. Your doctor, nurse, or pharmacist can help you avoid products that may cause a problem.

—if you are **pregnant** or if you may become pregnant. When hydrochlorothiazide is used during pregnancy, it may cause side effects including jaundice, blood problems, and low potassium in the newborn infant. Studies with hydralazine have not been done in humans. However, studies in mice have shown that hydralazine causes birth defects (cleft palate, defects in head and face bones); these birth defects may also occur in rabbits, but do not occur in rats.

—if you are **breast-feeding**. Hydrochlorothiazide passes into breast milk. However, neither hydralazine nor hydrochlorothiazide has been shown to cause problems in nursing babies.

—if you have any of the following medical problems:
  Diabetes mellitus (sugar diabetes)
  Gout
  Heart or blood vessel disease
  Kidney disease
  Liver disease
  Lupus erythematosus (history of)
  Pancreatitis (inflammation of the pancreas)

—if you have recently had a stroke.

—if you are taking **any** other prescription or nonprescription (OTC) medicine, especially one that contains:
  Adrenocorticoids (cortisone-like medicine)
  Diazoxide (e.g., Proglycem)
  Digitalis glycosides (heart medicine)
  Lithium (e.g., Lithane)
  Methenamine (e.g., Mandelamine)

Proper Use of This Medicine

This medicine may cause you to have an unusual feeling of tiredness when you begin to take it. You may also notice an increase in the amount of urine or in your frequency of urination. After taking the medicine for a while, these effects should lessen. To keep the increase in urine from affecting your nighttime sleep:

• If you are to take a single dose a day, take it in the morning after breakfast.

• If you are to take more than one dose a day, take the last dose no later than 6 p.m., unless otherwise directed by your doctor.

However, it is best to plan your dose or doses according to a schedule that will least affect your personal activities and sleep. Ask your doctor, nurse, or pharmacist to help you plan the best time to take this medicine.

Importance of diet—When prescribing medicine for your condition, your doctor may also prescribe a personal diet for you. Such a diet may be low in sodium (salt). Most people eat much more sodium than they need and too much sodium in the diet may increase blood pressure. Some foods that contain large amounts of sodium are canned soup, pickles, ketchup, green and ripe olives, relish, frankfurters, soy sauce, and carbonated beverages. Your doctor may want you to limit the amounts of these and other high-sodium foods in your diet. High blood pressure medicine is usually more effective when such a diet is properly followed.

Also, it may be very important for you to go on a reducing diet. However, check with your doctor before changing your diet.

Many patients who have high blood pressure will not notice any signs of the problem. In fact, many may feel normal. It is very important that you **take your medicine exactly as directed** and that you keep your appointments with your doctor even if you feel well.

Remember that this medicine will not cure your high blood pressure but it does help control it. Therefore, you must continue to take it as directed if you expect to lower your blood pressure and keep it down. **You may have to take high blood pressure medicine for the rest of your life.** If high blood pressure is not treated, it can cause serious problems such as heart failure, blood vessel disease, stroke, or kidney disease.

To help you remember to take your medicine, try to get into the habit of taking it at the same time each day.

If you miss a dose of this medicine, take it as soon as possible. However, if it is almost time for your next dose, skip the missed dose and go back to your regular dosing schedule. Do not double doses.

How to store this medicine:

- **Keep out of the reach of children.**

- Store away from heat and direct light.

- Do not store in the bathroom, near the kitchen sink, or in other damp places. Heat or moisture may cause the medicine to break down.

- Do not keep outdated medicine or medicine no longer needed. Be sure that any discarded medicine is out of the reach of children.

Precautions While Using This Medicine

It is important that your doctor check your progress at regular visits to make sure that this medicine is working properly.

Do not take other medicines unless they have been discussed with your doctor. This especially includes over-the-counter (nonprescription) medicines for appetite control, asthma, colds, cough, hay fever, or sinus problems, since they may tend to increase your blood pressure.

This medicine may cause some people to have headaches or to feel dizzy. **Make sure you know how you react to this medicine before you drive, use machines, or do other jobs that could be dangerous if you are not alert.**

Dizziness, lightheadedness, or fainting may occur, especially when you get up from a lying or sitting position. Getting up slowly may help, but if the problem continues or gets worse, check with your doctor.

The dizziness, lightheadedness, or fainting is also more likely to occur if you drink alcohol, stand for a long time, exercise, or if the weather is hot. **While you are taking this medicine, be careful in the amount of alcohol you drink. Also, use extra care during exercise or hot weather or if you must stand for a long time.**

This medicine may cause a loss of potassium from your body.

- To help prevent this, your doctor may want you to:
  —eat or drink foods that have a high potassium content (for example, orange or other citrus fruit juices), or

—take a potassium supplement, or

—take another medicine to help prevent the loss of the potassium in the first place.

• It is very important to follow these directions. Also, it is important not to change your diet on your own. This is more important if you are already on a special diet (as for diabetes), or if you are taking a potassium supplement or a medicine to reduce potassium loss. Extra potassium may not be necessary and, in some cases, too much potassium could be harmful.

Check with your doctor if you become sick and have severe or continuing nausea, vomiting, or diarrhea. These problems may cause you to lose additional water and potassium.

For diabetic patients:

• Thiazide diuretics may raise blood sugar levels. While you are using this medicine, be especially careful in testing for sugar in your blood or urine. If you have any questions about this, check with your doctor.

Some people who take this medicine may become more sensitive to sunlight than they are normally. **When you first begin taking this medicine, avoid too much sun and do not use a sunlamp until you see how you react to the sun,** especially if you tend to burn easily. **If you have a severe reaction, check with your doctor.**

Side Effects of This Medicine

Along with its needed effects, a medicine may cause some unwanted effects. Although not all of these side effects may occur, if they do occur they may need medical attention.

Check with your doctor as soon as possible if any of the following side effects occur:

Less common

Blisters on skin
Chest pain
General feeling of body discomfort or weakness
Joint pain

Numbness, tingling, pain, or weakness in hands or feet
Skin rash or itching
Sore throat and fever
Swelling of the lymph glands

Rare

Flank or stomach pain
Severe stomach pain with nausea and vomiting
Unusual bleeding or bruising
Yellow eyes or skin

Signs and symptoms of too much potassium loss

Dryness of mouth
Increased thirst
Irregular heartbeats
Mood or mental changes
Muscle cramps or pain
Weak pulse

Other side effects may occur that usually do not require
medical attention. These side effects may go away
during treatment as your body adjusts to the medicine.
However, check with your doctor if any of the following side effects continue or are bothersome:

More common

Decreased sexual ability
Diarrhea
Fast or irregular heartbeat
Headache
Loss of appetite
Nausea or vomiting

Less common

Dizziness or lightheadedness, especially when getting up from
a lying or sitting position
Increased sensitivity of skin to sunlight
Redness or flushing of the face
Shortness of breath with exercise or work
Stuffy nose
Watering or irritated eyes

For elderly patients:

• Some medicines may affect older patients differently than they do younger adults. Dizziness or lightheadedness or symptoms of too much potassium loss
may be more likely to occur in the elderly, who are

usually more sensitive to the effects of this medicine. Also, this medicine may reduce tolerance to cold temperatures in elderly patients. Check with your doctor if these occur. In addition, it is a good idea to check with your doctor or pharmacist if you notice any other unusual effects while taking this medicine or if you think it is not working as it should.

Other side effects not listed above may also occur in some patients. If you notice any other effects, check with your doctor.

INDAPAMIDE (Systemic)

Some commonly used brand names are:

In the U.S.
> Lozol

In Canada
> Lozide

Indapamide (in-DAP-a-mide) belongs to the group of medicines known as diuretics. It is commonly used to treat high blood pressure.

High blood pressure adds to the workload of the heart and arteries. If it continues for a long time, the heart and arteries may not function properly. This can damage the blood vessels of the brain, heart, and kidneys resulting in a stroke, heart failure, or kidney failure. High blood pressure may also increase the risk of heart attacks. These problems may be less likely to occur if blood pressure is controlled.

Indapamide is also used to help reduce the amount of water in the body by increasing the flow of urine.

Indapamide is available only with your doctor's prescription.

Before Using This Medicine

To decide on the best treatment for your medical problem, your doctor should be told:

—if you have ever had any unusual or allergic reaction to indapamide, sulfonamides (sulfa drugs), or thiazide diuretics (other water pills).

—if you are on a low-salt, low-sugar, or any other special diet, or if you are allergic to any substance, such as foods, sulfites or other preservatives, or dyes. Most medicines contain more than their active ingredient. Your doctor, nurse, or pharmacist can help you avoid products that may cause a problem.

—if you are **pregnant** or if you may become pregnant. Studies have not been done in humans. However, indapamide has not been shown to cause birth defects or other problems in animal studies.

In general, diuretics are not useful for normal swelling of feet and hands that occurs during pregnancy. Diuretics should not be taken during pregnancy unless recommended by your doctor.

—if you are **breast-feeding**. It is not known whether indapamide passes into the breast milk. However, this medicine has not been shown to cause problems in nursing babies.

—if you have any of the following medical problems:
Diabetes mellitus (sugar diabetes)
Gout (history of)
Kidney disease
Liver disease

—if you are taking **any** other prescription or nonprescription (OTC) medicine, especially one that contains:
Adrenocorticoids (cortisone-like medicine)
Digitalis glycosides (heart medicine)
Lithium (e.g., Lithane)

Proper Use of This Medicine

Indapamide may cause you to have an unusual feeling of tiredness when you begin to take it. You may also notice an increase in the amount of urine or in your frequency of urination. After taking the medicine for a while, these effects should lessen. To keep the increase in urine from affecting your nighttime sleep:

• if you are to take a single dose a day, take it in the morning after breakfast.

• if you are to take more than one dose a day, take the last dose no later than 6 p.m., unless otherwise directed by your doctor.

However, it is best to plan your dose or doses according to a schedule that will least affect your personal activities and sleep. Ask your doctor, nurse, or pharmacist to help you plan the best time to take this medicine.

To help you remember to take indapamide, try to get into the habit of taking it at the same time each day.

For patients taking indapamide for high blood pressure:
• Importance of diet—When prescribing medicine for your condition your doctor may also prescribe a personal

diet for you. Such a diet may be low in sodium (salt). Most people eat much more sodium than they need. Too much sodium in the diet may increase blood pressure. Some foods that contain large amounts of sodium are canned soup, pickles, ketchup, green and ripe olives, relish, frankfurters, soy sauce, and carbonated beverages. Your doctor may want you to limit the amounts of these and other high-sodium foods in your diet. High blood pressure medicine is usually more effective when such a diet is properly followed.

Also, it may be very important for you to go on a reducing diet. However, check with your doctor before changing your diet.

• Many patients who have high blood pressure will not notice any signs of the problem. In fact, many may feel normal. It is very important that you **take your medicine exactly as directed** and that you keep your appointments with your doctor even if you feel well.

• Remember that this medicine will not cure your high blood pressure but it does help control it. Therefore, you must continue to take it as directed if you expect to lower your blood pressure and keep it down. **You may have to take high blood pressure medicine for the rest of your life.** If high blood pressure is not treated, it can cause serious problems such as heart failure, blood vessel disease, stroke, or kidney disease.

If you miss a dose of this medicine, take it as soon as possible. However, if it is almost time for your next dose, skip the missed dose and go back to your regular dosing schedule. Do not double doses.

How to store this medicine:

• **Keep out of the reach of children.**

• Store away from heat and direct light.

• Do not store in the bathroom, near the kitchen sink, or in other damp places. Heat or moisture may cause the medicine to break down.

• Do not keep outdated medicine or medicine no longer needed. Be sure that any discarded medicine is out of the reach of children.

Precautions While Using This Medicine

It is important that your doctor check your progress at regular visits to make sure that indapamide is working properly.

This medicine may cause a loss of potassium from your body:

- To help prevent this, your doctor may want you to:

  —eat or drink foods that have a high potassium content (for example, orange or other citrus fruit juices), or

  —take a potassium supplement, or

  —take another medication to help prevent the loss of the potassium in the first place.

- It is very important to follow these directions. Also, it is important not to change your diet on your own. This is more important if you are already on a special diet (as for diabetes), or if you are taking a potassium supplement or a medicine to reduce potassium loss. Extra potassium may not be necessary and, in some cases, too much potassium could be harmful.

Check with your doctor if you become sick and have severe or continuing vomiting or diarrhea. These problems may cause you to lose additional water and potassium.

For patients taking this medicine for high blood pressure:

- **Do not take other medicines unless they have been discussed with your doctor.** This especially includes over-the-counter (nonprescription) medicines for appetite control, asthma, colds, hay fever, or sinus problems, since they may tend to increase your blood pressure.

Side Effects of This Medicine

Along with its needed effects, a medicine may cause some unwanted effects. Although not all of these side effects may occur, if they do occur they may need medical attention.

Check with your doctor as soon as possible if any of the following side effects occur:

Signs and symptoms of too much potassium loss
    Dryness of mouth

Increased thirst
Irregular heartbeat
Mood or mental changes
Muscle cramps or pain
Nausea or vomiting
Unusual tiredness or weakness
Weak pulse

Rare

Skin rash, itching, or hives

Other side effects may occur that usually do not require medical attention. These side effects may go away during treatment as your body adjusts to the medicine. However, check with your doctor if any of the following side effects continue or are bothersome:

Less common or rare

Diarrhea
Dizziness or lightheadedness, especially when getting up from a lying or sitting position
Headache
Loss of appetite
Trouble in sleeping
Upset stomach

For elderly patients:

• Some medicines may affect older patients differently than they do younger adults. Dizziness or lightheadedness and signs and symptoms of too much potassium loss are more likely to occur in the elderly, who are usually more sensitive to the effects of indapamide. Check with your doctor if these occur. In addition, it is a good idea to check with your doctor or pharmacist if you notice any other unusual effects while taking this medicine or if you think it is not working as it should.

Other side effects not listed above may also occur in some patients. If you notice any other effects, check with your doctor.

MECAMYLAMINE (Systemic)

A commonly used brand name in the U.S. is Inversine.

Mecamylamine (mek-a-MILL-a-meen) belongs to the general class of medicines called antihypertensives. It is taken by mouth to treat high blood pressure.

High blood pressure adds to the workload of the heart and arteries. If it continues for a long time, the heart and arteries may not function properly. This can damage the blood vessels of the brain, heart, and kidneys, resulting in a stroke, heart failure, or kidney failure. High blood pressure may also increase the risk of heart attacks. These problems may be less likely to occur if blood pressure is controlled.

Mecamylamine works by controlling impulses along certain nerve pathways. As a result, it relaxes blood vessels so that blood passes through them more easily. This helps to lower blood pressure.

Mecamylamine is available only with your doctor's prescription.

Before Using This Medicine

To decide on the best treatment for your medical problem, your doctor should be told:

—if you have ever had any unusual or allergic reaction to mecamylamine.

—if you are on a low-salt, low-sugar, or any other special diet, or if you are allergic to any substance, such as foods, sulfites or other preservatives, or dyes. Most medicines contain more than their active ingredient. Your doctor, nurse, or pharmacist can help you avoid products that may cause a problem.

—if you are **pregnant** or if you may become pregnant. Mecamylamine may cause bowel problems in the fetus. This medicine has not been shown to cause birth defects. However, in general, use of this medicine during pregnancy is not recommended because pregnant women may be more sensitive to its effects.

—if you are **breast-feeding**. This medicine has not been shown to cause problems in nursing babies.

—if you have any of the following medical problems:
Bladder or prostate problems
Bowel problems
Diarrhea
Fever or infection
Glaucoma
Gout
Heart or blood vessel disease
Kidney disease
Nausea or vomiting

—if you have recently had a heart attack or stroke.

—if you are taking **any** other prescription or nonprescription (OTC) medicine, especially one that contains:
Antibiotics
Sulfonamides (sulfa medicine)
Urinary alkalizers (medicine that makes the urine less acid, such as acetazolamide [e.g., Diamox], calcium- and/or magnesium-containing antacids, dichlorphenamide [e.g., Daranide], methazolamide [e.g., Neptazane], potassium or sodium citrate and/or citric acid, sodium bicarbonate [baking soda])

Proper Use of This Medicine

Importance of diet—When prescribing medicine for your condition, your doctor may also prescribe a personal diet for you. Such a diet may be low in sodium (salt). Most people eat much more sodium than they need and too much sodium in the diet may increase blood pressure. Some foods that contain large amounts of sodium are canned soup, pickles, ketchup, green and ripe olives, relish, frankfurters, soy sauce, and carbonated beverages. Your doctor may want you to limit the amounts of these and other high-sodium foods in your diet. High blood pressure medicine is usually more effective when such a diet is properly followed.

Also, it may be very important for you to go on a reducing diet. However, check with your doctor before changing your diet.

Many patients who have high blood pressure will not notice any signs of the problem. In fact, many may feel normal. **It is very important that you take your medicine exactly**

as directed and that you keep your appointments with your doctor even if you feel well.

Remember that this medicine will not cure your high blood pressure but it does help control it. Therefore, you must continue to take it as directed if you expect to lower your blood pressure and keep it down. **You may have to take high blood pressure medicine for the rest of your life.** If high blood pressure is not treated, it can cause serious problems such as heart failure, blood vessel disease, stroke, or kidney disease.

To help you remember to take your medicine, try to get into the habit of taking it at the same time each day.

If you do miss a dose of this medicine, take it as soon as possible. Then go back to your regular dosing schedule. **If you miss two or more doses in a row, check with your doctor right away.** If your body goes without this medicine for too long, your blood pressure may go up to a dangerously high level.

How to store this medicine:

- **Keep out of the reach of children.**

- Store away from heat and direct light.

- Do not store in the bathroom, near the kitchen sink, or in other damp places. Heat or moisture may cause the medicine to break down.

- Do not keep outdated medicine or medicine no longer needed. Be sure that any discarded medicine is out of the reach of children.

Precautions While Using This Medicine

It is important that your doctor check your progress at regular visits to make sure that this medicine is working properly.

Check with your doctor before you stop taking this medicine. Your doctor may want you to reduce gradually the amount you are taking before stopping completely.

Make sure that you have enough medicine on hand to last through weekends, holidays, or vacations. You should not

miss taking any doses. You may want to ask your doctor
for another written prescription for mecamylamine to carry
in your wallet or purse. You can then have it filled if you
run out of medicine when you are away from home.

**Do not take other medicines unless they have been discussed
with your doctor.** This especially includes over-the-counter
(nonprescription) medicines for appetite control, asthma,
colds, cough, hay fever, or sinus problems, since they may
tend to increase your blood pressure.

**Dizziness, lightheadedness, or fainting may occur, especially
when you get up from a lying or sitting position.** This is
more likely to occur in the morning. **Getting up slowly
may help.** When you get up from lying down, sit on the
edge of the bed with your feet dangling for one or two
minutes. Then stand up slowly. If you feel dizzy, sit or
lie down. If the problem continues or gets worse, check
with your doctor.

The dizziness, lightheadedness, or fainting is also more likely
to occur if you drink alcohol, stand for a long time, exercise, or if the weather is hot. **While you are taking this
medicine, be careful in the amount of alcohol you drink.
Also, use extra care during exercise or hot weather or if
you must stand for a long time.**

Sodium bicarbonate (commonly known as baking soda) may
cause you to get a greater than normal effect from this
medicine. To prevent problems, check with your doctor
or pharmacist before using an antacid or medicine for
heartburn since some of these contain sodium bicarbonate.

Tell your doctor if you get a fever or infection since that
may change the amount of medicine you have to take.

Mecamylamine may cause dryness of the mouth, nose, and
throat. For temporary relief of mouth dryness, use sugarless candy or gum, melt bits of ice in your mouth, or
use a saliva substitute. However, if dry mouth continues
for more than 2 weeks, check with your physician or
dentist. Continuing dryness of the mouth may increase

the chance of dental disease, including tooth decay, gum disease, and fungus infections.

Before having any kind of surgery (including dental surgery) or emergency treatment, tell the physician or dentist in charge that you are taking this medicine.

Side Effects of This Medicine

Along with its needed effects, a medicine may cause some unwanted effects. Although not all of these side effects may occur, if they do occur they may need medical attention.

Check with your doctor as soon as possible if any of the following side effects occur:

More common

Dizziness or lightheadedness, especially when getting up from a lying or sitting position

Less common

Difficult urination

Rare

Confusion or excitement
Mental depression
Shortness of breath
Trembling

Other side effects may occur that usually do not require medical attention. These side effects may go away during treatment as your body adjusts to the medicine. However, check with your doctor if any of the following side effects continue or are bothersome:

More common

Constipation
Drowsiness
Unusual tiredness

Less common or rare

Blurred vision
Decreased sexual ability
Dry mouth
Enlarged pupils
Loss of appetite

Nausea and vomiting
Weakness

For elderly patients:

• Some medicines may affect older patients differently than they do younger adults. Dizziness or light-headedness may be more likely to occur in the elderly, who are more sensitive to the effects of mecamylamine. Check with your doctor if this occurs. In addition, it is good idea to check with your doctor or pharmacist if you notice any other unusual effects while taking this medicine or if you think it is not working as it should.

Other side effects not listed above may also occur in some patients. If you notice any other effects, check with your doctor.

METHYLDOPA (Systemic)

Some commonly used brand names are:

In the U.S.
    Aldomet

    Generic name product may also be available.

In Canada
    Aldomet   Dopamet
    Apo-Methyldopa   Novomedopa

    Generic name product may also be available.

Methyldopa (meth-ill-DOE-pa) belongs to the general class of medicines called antihypertensives. It is used to treat high blood pressure.

High blood pressure adds to the workload of the heart and arteries. If it continues for a long time, the heart and arteries may not function properly. This can damage the blood vessels of the brain, heart, and kidneys, resulting in a stroke, heart failure, or kidney failure. High blood pressure may also increase the risk of heart attacks. These problems may be less likely to occur if blood pressure is controlled.

Methyldopa works by controlling impulses along certain nerve pathways. As a result, it relaxes blood vessels so that blood passes through them more easily. This helps to lower blood pressure.

Methyldopa is available only with your doctor's prescription.

Before Using This Medicine

To decide on the best treatment for your medical problem, your doctor should be told:

—if you have ever had any unusual or allergic reaction to methyldopa.

—if you are on a low-salt, low-sugar, or any other special diet, or if you are allergic to any substance, such as foods, sulfites or other preservatives, or dyes. Most medicines contain more than their active ingredient and some methyldopa products may contain sulfites. Your doctor, nurse, or pharmacist can help you avoid products that may cause a problem.

—if you are **pregnant** or if you may become pregnant. Studies in humans have not shown that methyldopa causes birth defects or other problems.

—if you are **breast-feeding**. Although methyldopa passes into breast milk, it has not been shown to cause problems in nursing babies.

—if you have any of the following medical problems:
Angina (chest pain)
Kidney disease
Liver disease
Mental depression (history of)
Parkinson's disease
Pheochromocytoma (PCC)

—if you have taken methyldopa in the past and developed liver problems.

—if you are now taking or have taken within the past 2 weeks monoamine oxidase (MAO) inhibitors, such as:
Furazolidone (e.g., Furoxone)
Isocarboxazid (e.g., Marplan)
Pargyline (e.g., Eutonyl)
Phenelzine (e.g., Nardil)
Procarbazine (e.g., Matulane)
Tranylcypromine (e.g., Parnate)

—if you are taking **any** other prescription or nonprescription (OTC) medicine.

Proper Use of This Medicine

Importance of diet—When prescribing medicine for your condition, your doctor may also prescribe a personal diet for you. Such a diet may be low in sodium (salt). Most people eat much more sodium than they need and too much sodium in the diet may increase blood pressure. Some foods that contain large amounts of sodium are canned soup, pickles, ketchup, green and ripe olives, relish, frankfurters, soy sauce, and carbonated beverages. Your doctor may want you to limit the amounts of these and other high-sodium foods in your diet. High blood pressure medicine is usually more effective when such a diet is properly followed.

Also, it may be very important for you to go on a reducing diet. However, check with your doctor before changing your diet.

Many patients who have high blood pressure will not notice any signs of the problem. In fact, many may feel normal.

It is very important that you **take your medicine exactly as directed** and that you keep your appointments with your doctor even if you feel well.

Remember that methyldopa will not cure your high blood pressure but it does help control it. Therefore, you must continue to take it as directed if you expect to lower your blood pressure and keep it down. **You may have to take high blood pressure medicine for the rest of your life.** If high blood pressure is not treated, it can cause serious problems such as heart failure, blood vessel disease, stroke, or kidney disease.

To help you remember to take your medicine, try to get into the habit of taking it at the same time each day.

If you miss a dose of this medicine, take it as soon as possible. However, if it is almost time for your next dose, skip the missed dose and go back to your regular dosing schedule. Do not double doses.

How to store this medicine:

- **Keep out of the reach of children.**

- Store away from heat and direct light.

- Do not store in the bathroom, near the kitchen sink, or in other damp places. Heat or moisture may cause the medicine to break down.

- Keep the oral liquid form of this medicine from freezing.

- Do not keep outdated medicine or medicine no longer needed. Be sure that any discarded medicine is out of the reach of children.

Precautions While Using This Medicine

It is important that your doctor check your progress at regular visits to make sure that this medicine is working properly.

Do not take other medicines unless they have been discussed with your doctor. This especially includes over-the-counter (nonprescription) medicines for appetite control, asthma, colds, cough, hay fever, or sinus problems, since they may tend to increase your blood pressure.

If you have a fever and there seems to be no reason for it, check with your doctor. This is especially important during the first few weeks you take methyldopa, since fever may be a sign of a serious reaction to this medicine.

Before having any kind of surgery (including dental surgery) or emergency treatment, make sure the physician or dentist in charge knows that you are taking this medicine.

Methyldopa may cause some people to become drowsy or less alert than they are normally. This is more likely to happen when you begin to take it or when you increase the amount of medicine you are taking. **Make sure you know how you react to this medicine before you drive, use machines, or do other jobs that could be dangerous if you are not alert.**

Dizziness, lightheadedness, or fainting may occur, especially when you get up from a lying or sitting position. Getting up slowly may help, but if the problem continues or gets worse, check with your doctor.

Methyldopa may cause dryness of the mouth. For temporary relief, use sugarless candy or gum, melt bits of ice in your mouth, or use a saliva substitute. However, if dry mouth continues for more than 2 weeks, check with your physician or dentist. Continuing dryness of the mouth may increase the chance of dental disease, including tooth decay, gum disease, and fungus infections.

Tell the doctor in charge that you are taking this medicine before you have any medical tests. The results of some tests may be affected by this medicine.

Side Effects of This Medicine

Along with its needed effects, a medicine may cause some unwanted effects. Although not all of these side effects may occur, if they do occur they may need medical attention.

Check with your doctor immediately if the following side effect occurs:

Less common

Fever shortly after starting to take this medicine

Check with your doctor as soon as possible if any of the following side effects occur:

More common

Swelling of feet or lower legs

Less common

Mental depression or anxiety
Nightmares or unusually vivid dreams
Trouble in sleeping

Rare

Dark or amber urine
Diarrhea or stomach cramps (severe or continuing)
Fever, chills, troubled breathing, and fast heartbeat
Pale stools
Shakiness or unusual body movements
Sore throat and fever
Stomach pain (severe) with nausea and vomiting
Tiredness or weakness after having taken this medicine for
    several weeks (continuing)
Unusual bleeding or bruising
Yellow eyes or skin

Other side effects may occur that usually do not require medical attention. These side effects may go away during treatment as your body adjusts to the medicine. However, check with your doctor if any of the following side effects continue or are bothersome:

More common

Drowsiness
Dry mouth
Headache

Less common

Decreased sexual ability
Diarrhea
Dizziness or lightheadedness when getting up from a lying
    or sitting position
Fainting
Nausea or vomiting

Numbness, tingling, pain, or weakness in hands or feet
Skin rash
Slow heartbeat
Stuffy nose
Swelling of the breasts or unusual milk production

For elderly patients:

• Some medicines may affect older patients differently than they do younger adults. Dizziness or lightheadedness and drowsiness may be more likely to occur in the elderly, who are more sensitive to the effects of methyldopa. Check with your doctor if these continue or are bothersome. In addition, it is a good idea to check with your doctor or pharmacist if you notice any other unusual effects while taking this medicine or if you think it is not working as it should.

Other side effects not listed above may also occur in some patients. If you notice any other effects, check with your doctor.

METHYLDOPA AND THIAZIDE DIURETICS (Systemic)

This information applies to the following medicines:

Methyldopa (meth-ill-DOE-pa) and Chlorothiazide (klor-oh-THYE-a-zide)
Methyldopa and Hydrochlorothiazide (hye-droe-klor-oh-THYE-a-zide)

Some commonly used brand names are:

For Methyldopa and Chlorothiazide
In the U.S.
Aldoclor

Generic name product may also be available.

In Canada
Supres

For Methyldopa and Hydrochlorothiazide
In the U.S.
Aldoril

Generic name product may also be available.

In Canada
Aldoril   PMS Dopazide
Novodoparil

Combinations of methyldopa and a thiazide diuretic (chlorothiazide or hydrochlorothiazide) are taken by mouth to treat high blood pressure.

High blood pressure adds to the workload of the heart and arteries. If it continues for a long time, the heart and arteries may not function properly. This can damage the blood vessels of the brain, heart, and kidneys, resulting in a stroke, heart failure, or kidney failure. High blood pressure may also increase the risk of heart attacks. These problems may be less likely to occur if blood pressure is controlled.

Methyldopa works by controlling nerve impulses along certain nerve pathways. As a result, it relaxes blood vessels so that blood passes through them more easily. Thiazide diuretics help reduce the amount of water in the body by increasing the flow of urine. These actions help to lower blood pressure.

This medicine is available only with your doctor's prescription.

Before Using This Medicine

To decide on the best treatment for your medical problem, your doctor should be told:

—if you have ever had any unusual or allergic reaction to methyldopa, sulfonamides (sulfa drugs), indapamide, or thiazide diuretics (water pills).

—if you are on a low-salt, low-sugar, or any other special diet, or if you are allergic to any substance, such as foods, sulfites or other preservatives, or dyes. Most medicines contain more than their active ingredient. Your doctor, nurse, or pharmacist can help you avoid products that may cause a problem.

—if you are **pregnant** or if you may become pregnant. Studies in humans have not shown that methyldopa causes birth defects or other problems. However, when thiazide diuretics are used during pregnancy, they may cause side effects including jaundice, blood problems, and low potassium in the newborn infant. Thiazide diuretics have not been shown to cause birth defects.

—if you are **breast-feeding**. Although this medicine passes into breast milk, it has not been shown to cause problems in nursing babies.

—if you have any of the following medical problems:
  Angina (chest pain)
  Diabetes mellitus (sugar diabetes)
  Gout (history of)
  Kidney disease
  Liver disease
  Lupus erythematosus (history of)
  Mental depression (history of)
  Pancreatitis (inflammation of the pancreas)
  Parkinson's disease
  Pheochromocytoma (PCC)

—if you have taken methyldopa in the past and developed liver problems.

—if you are now taking or have taken within the past 2 weeks monoamine oxidase (MAO) inhibitors, such as:
  Furazolidone (e.g., Furoxone)
  Isocarboxazid (e.g., Marplan)
  Pargyline (e.g., Eutonyl)
  Phenelzine (e.g., Nardil)
  Procarbazine (e.g., Matulane)
  Tranylcypromine (e.g., Parnate)

—if you are taking **any** other prescription or nonprescription (OTC) medicine, especially one that contains:

Adrenocorticoids (cortisone-like medicines)
Digitalis glycosides (heart medicine)
Lithium (e.g., Lithane)
Methenamine (e.g., Mandelamine)

Proper Use of This Medicine

Importance of diet—When prescribing medicine for your condition, your doctor may also prescribe a personal diet for you. Such a diet may be low in sodium (salt). Most people eat much more sodium than they need and too much sodium in the diet may increase blood pressure. Some foods that contain large amounts of sodium are canned soup, pickles, ketchup, green and ripe olives, relish, frankfurters, soy sauce, and carbonated beverages. Your doctor may want you to limit the amounts of these and other high-sodium foods in your diet. High blood pressure medicine is usually more effective when such a diet is properly followed.

Also, it may be very important for you to go on a reducing diet. However, check with your doctor before changing your diet.

Many patients who have high blood pressure will not notice any signs of the problem. In fact, many may feel normal. It is very important **that you take your medicine exactly as directed** and that you keep your appointments with your doctor even if you feel well.

Remember that this medicine will not cure your high blood pressure but it does help control it. Therefore, you must continue to take it as directed if you expect to lower your blood pressure and keep it down. **You may have to take high blood pressure medicine for the rest of your life.** If high blood pressure is not treated, it can cause serious problems such as heart failure, blood vessel disease, stroke, or kidney disease.

This medicine may cause you to have an unusual feeling of tiredness when you begin to take it. You may also notice an increase in the amount of urine or in your frequency of urination. After taking the medicine for a while, these effects should lessen. In general, to keep the increase in urine from affecting your sleep:

• If you are to take a single dose a day, take it in the morning after breakfast.

• If you are to take more than one dose a day, take the last dose no later than 6 p.m., unless otherwise directed by your doctor.

However, it is best to plan your dose or doses according to a schedule that will least affect your personal activities and sleep. Ask your doctor, nurse, or pharmacist to help you plan the best time to take this medicine.

To help you remember to take your medicine, try to get into the habit of taking it at the same time each day.

If you miss a dose of this medicine, take it as soon as possible. However, if it is almost time for your next dose, skip the missed dose and go back to your regular dosing schedule. Do not double doses.

How to store this medicine:

• **Keep out of the reach of children.**

• Store away from heat and direct light.

• Do not store in the bathroom, near the kitchen sink, or in other damp places. Heat or moisture may cause the medicine to break down.

• Do not keep outdated medicine or medicine no longer needed. Be sure that any discarded medicine is out of the reach of children.

Precautions While Using This Medicine

It is important that your doctor check your progress at regular visits to make sure that this medicine is working properly.

Do not take other medicines unless they have been discussed with your doctor. This especially includes over-the-counter (nonprescription) medicines for appetite control, asthma, colds, cough, hay fever, or sinus problems, since they may tend to increase your blood pressure.

This medicine may cause a loss of potassium from your body:

- To help prevent this, your doctor may want you to:

  —eat or drink foods that have a high potassium content (for example, orange or other citrus fruit juices), or

  —take a potassium supplement, or

  —take another medicine to help prevent the loss of the potassium in the first place.

- It is very important to follow these directions. Also, it is important not to change your diet on your own. This is more important if you are already on a special diet (as for diabetes), or if you are taking a potassium supplement or a medicine to reduce potassium loss. Extra potassium may not be necessary and, in some cases, too much potassium could be harmful.

Check with your doctor if you become sick and have severe or continuing vomiting or diarrhea. These problems may cause you to lose additional water and potassium.

Before having any kind of surgery (including dental surgery) or emergency treatment, tell the physician or dentist in charge that you are taking this medicine.

If you have a fever and there seems to be no reason for it, check with your doctor. This is especially important during the first few weeks you take this medicine since fever may be a sign of a serious reaction to methyldopa.

This medicine may cause some people to become drowsy or less alert than they are normally. This is more likely to happen when you begin to take it or when you increase the amount of medicine you are taking. **Make sure you know how you react to this medicine before you drive, use machines, or do other jobs that could be dangerous if you are not alert.**

Dizziness, lightheadedness, or fainting may occur, especially when you get up from a lying or sitting position. Getting up slowly may help, but if the problem continues or gets worse, check with your doctor.

The dizziness, lightheadedness, or fainting is also more likely to occur if you drink alcohol, stand for long periods of time, exercise, or if the weather is hot. Drinking alcoholic beverages may also make the drowsiness worse. **While you are taking this medicine, be careful in the amount of alcohol you drink.** Also, use extra care during exercise or hot weather or if you must stand for long periods of time.

For diabetic patients:

• This medicine may raise blood sugar levels. While you are using this medicine, be especially careful in testing for sugar in your urine. If you have any questions about this, check with your doctor.

This medicine may cause dryness of the mouth. For temporary relief, use sugarless candy or gum, melt bits of ice in your mouth, or use a saliva substitute. However, if dry mouth continues for more than 2 weeks, check with your physician or dentist. Continuing dryness of the mouth may increase the chance of dental disease, including tooth decay, gum disease, and fungus infections.

A few people who take this medicine may become more sensitive to sunlight than they are normally. **When you first begin taking this medicine, avoid too much sun and do not use a sunlamp until you see how you react to the sun,** especially if you tend to burn easily. **If you have a severe reaction, check with your doctor.**

Tell the doctor in charge that you are taking this medicine before you have any medical tests. The results of some tests may be affected by this medicine.

Side Effects of This Medicine

Along with its needed effects, a medicine may cause some unwanted effects. Although not all of these side effects may occur, if they do occur they may need medical attention.

Check with your doctor immediately if the following side effect occurs:

Rare

Unexplained fever shortly after starting to take this medicine

Check with your doctor as soon as possible if any of the following side effects occur, especially since some of them may mean that your body is losing too much potassium:

Signs and symptoms of too much potassium loss

Dryness of mouth
Increased thirst
Irregular heartbeats
Muscle cramps or pain
Nausea or vomiting
Unusual tiredness or weakness
Weak pulse

Less common

Mental depression or anxiety
Nightmares or unusually vivid dreams
Trouble in sleeping

Rare

Dark or amber urine
Diarrhea or stomach cramps (severe or continuing)
Fever, chills, troubled breathing, and fast heartbeat
Joint pain
Lower back, side, or stomach pain
Pale stools
Shakiness or unusual body movements
Skin rash or hives
Stomach pain (severe) with nausea and vomiting
Tiredness or weakness after having taken this medicine for
     several weeks (continuing)
Unusual bleeding or bruising
Yellow eyes or skin

Other side effects may occur that usually do not require medical attention. These side effects may go away during treatment as your body adjusts to the medicine. However, check with your doctor if any of the following side effects continue or are bothersome:

More common

Dizziness or lightheadedness when getting up from a lying
     or sitting position
Drowsiness
Headache

Less common
    Decreased sexual ability
    Diarrhea
    Fainting
    Increased sensitivity to sunlight
    Loss of appetite
    Numbness, tingling, pain, or weakness in hands or feet
    Skin rash
    Slow heartbeat
    Stuffy nose
    Swelling of the breasts or unusual milk production

For elderly patients:

• Some medicines may affect older patients differently than they do younger adults. Dizziness or lightheadedness, drowsiness, or signs of too much potassium loss may be more likely to occur in the elderly, who are more sensitive to the effects of methyldopa and thiazide diuretics. Check with your doctor if these occur. In addition, it is a good idea to check with your doctor or pharmacist if you notice any other unusual effects while taking this medicine or if you think it is not working as it should.

Other side effects not listed above may also occur in some patients. If you notice any other effects, check with your doctor.

METYROSINE (Systemic)

A commonly used brand name in the U.S. is Demser.

Metyrosine (me-TYE-roe-seen) belongs to the general class of medicines called antihypertensives. It is taken by mouth to treat high blood pressure caused by a disease called pheochromocytoma.

Metyrosine reduces the amount of certain chemicals in the body. When these chemicals are present in large amounts, they cause high blood pressure.

Metyrosine is available only with your doctor's prescription.

Before Using This Medicine

To decide on the best treatment for your medical problem, your doctor should be told:

—if you have ever had any unusual or allergic reaction to metyrosine.

—if you are on a low-salt, low-sugar, or any other special diet, or if you are allergic to any substance, such as foods, sulfites or other preservatives, or dyes. Most medicines contain more than their active ingredient. Your doctor, nurse, or pharmacist can help you avoid products that may cause a problem.

—if you are **pregnant** or if you may become pregnant. Studies have not been done in either humans or animals.

—if you are **breast-feeding**. It is not known whether metyrosine passes into the breast milk. However, this medicine has not been shown to cause problems in nursing babies.

—if you have any of the following medical problems:
  Kidney disease
  Liver disease
  Mental depression (or history of)
  Parkinson's disease

—if you are taking **any** other prescription or nonprescription (OTC) medicine.

Proper Use of This Medicine

Take this medicine only as directed by your doctor. Do not take more or less of it than your doctor ordered.

To help you remember to take your medicine, try to get into the habit of taking it at the same times each day.

If you miss a dose of this medicine, take it as soon as possible. However, if it is almost time for your next dose, skip the missed dose and go back to your regular dosing schedule. Do not double doses.

How to store this medicine:

- **Keep out of the reach of children.**

- Store away from heat and direct light.

- Do not store in the bathroom, near the kitchen sink, or in other damp places. Heat or moisture may cause the medicine to break down.

- Do not keep outdated medicine or medicine no longer needed. Be sure that any discarded medicine is out of the reach of children.

Precautions While Using This Medicine

It is important that your doctor check your progress at regular visits to make sure that this medicine is working properly and to check for unwanted effects.

While taking this medicine, it is important that you drink plenty of fluids and urinate often. This will help prevent kidney problems and keep your kidneys working well. If you have any questions about how much you should drink, check with your doctor.

This medicine will add to the effects of alcohol and other CNS depressants (medicines that slow down the nervous system, possibly causing drowsiness). Some examples of CNS depressants are antihistamines or medicine for hay fever, other allergies, or colds; sedatives, tranquilizers, or sleeping medicine; prescription pain medicine or narcotics; barbiturates; medicine for seizures; tricyclic antidepressants (medicine for depression); muscle relaxants; or anesthetics, including some dental anesthetics. **Check with your doctor before taking any of the above while you are taking this medicine.**

Before having any kind of surgery (including dental surgery), tell the physician or dentist in charge that you are taking this medicine.

This medicine may cause most people to become drowsy or less alert than they are normally. **Make sure you know how you react to this medicine before you drive, use machines, or do other jobs that could be dangerous if you are not alert.**

Side Effects of This Medicine

Along with its needed effects, a medicine may cause some unwanted effects. Although not all of these side effects may occur, if they do occur they may need medical attention.

Check with your doctor as soon as possible if any of the following side effects occur:

More common

Diarrhea
Difficulty in speaking
Drooling
Trembling and shaking of hands and fingers

Less common

Anxiety
Confusion
Hallucinations (seeing, hearing, or feeling things that are not there)
Mental depression

Rare

Blood in urine
Decrease in urination
Muscle spasms, especially of neck and back
Painful urination
Restlessness
Shortness of breath
Shuffling walk
Skin rash and itching
Swelling of feet or lower legs
Tic-like (jerky) movements of head, face, mouth, and neck

Other side effects may occur that usually do not require medical attention. These side effects may go away during treatment as your body adjusts to the medicine. However, check with your doctor if the following side effect continues or is bothersome:

Drowsiness

For elderly patients:

• Many medicines have not been tested in older people. Therefore, it may not be known whether they work exactly the same way they do in younger adults or if they cause different side effects or problems in older people. There is no specific information about the use of metyrosine in the elderly. However, it is a good idea to check with your doctor or pharmacist if you notice any unusual effects while taking this medicine or if you think it is not working as it should.

After you stop taking this medicine, it may still produce some side effects that need attention. During this period of time check with your doctor if you notice the following side effect:

Diarrhea

Also, after you stop taking this medicine, you may have feelings of increased energy or you may have trouble in sleeping. However, these effects should last only for two or three days.

Other side effects not listed above may also occur in some patients. If you notice any other effects, check with your doctor.

MINOXIDIL (Systemic)

Some commonly used brand names are:

In the U.S.
        Loniten
        Minodyl
    Generic name product may also be available.

In Canada
        Loniten

Minoxidil (mi-NOX-i-dill) belongs to the general class of medicines called antihypertensives. It is taken by mouth to treat high blood pressure.

High blood pressure adds to the workload of the heart and arteries. If it continues for a long time, the heart and arteries may not function properly. This can damage the blood vessels of the brain, heart, and kidneys, resulting in a stroke, heart failure, or kidney failure. High blood pressure may also increase the risk of heart attacks. These problems may be less likely to occur if blood pressure is controlled.

Minoxidil works by relaxing blood vessels so that blood passes through them more easily. This helps to lower blood pressure.

Minoxidil has other effects that could be bothersome for some patients. These include increased hair growth, weight gain, fast heartbeat, and chest pain. Before you take this medicine, be sure that you have discussed the use of it with your doctor.

Minoxidil is being applied to the scalp in liquid form by some balding men to stimulate hair growth. However, improper use of liquids made from minoxidil tablets can result in minoxidil being absorbed into the body, where it may cause unwanted effects on the heart and blood vessels.

Minoxidil is available only with your doctor's prescription.

Before Using This Medicine

To decide on the best treatment for your medical problem, your doctor should be told:

—if you have ever had any unusual or allergic reaction to minoxidil.

—if you are on a low-salt, low-sugar, or any other special diet, or if you are allergic to any substance, such as foods, sulfites or other preservatives, or dyes. Most medicines contain more than their active ingredient. Your doctor, nurse, or pharmacist can help you avoid products that may cause a problem.

—if you are **pregnant** or if you may become pregnant. Studies have not been done in humans. However, studies in rats found a decreased rate of conception, and studies in rabbits at 5 times the human dose have shown a decrease in successful pregnancies. Minoxidil did not cause birth defects in rats or rabbits.

—if you are **breast-feeding**. Although minoxidil passes into breast milk, it has not been shown to cause problems in nursing babies.

—if you have any of the following medical problems:
Angina (chest pain)
Heart or blood vessel disease
Kidney disease
Pheochromocytoma

—if you have recently had a heart attack or stroke.

—if you are taking **any** other prescription or nonprescription (OTC) medicine, especially one that contains:
Guanethidine (e.g., Ismelin)
Nitrates (medicine for angina)

Proper Use of This Medicine

Importance of diet—When prescribing medicine for your condition, your doctor may also prescribe a personal diet for you. Such a diet may be low in sodium (salt). Most people eat much more sodium than they need and too much sodium in the diet may increase blood pressure. Some foods that contain large amounts of sodium are canned soup, pickles, ketchup, green and ripe olives, relish, frankfurters, soy sauce, and carbonated beverages. Your doctor may want you to limit the amounts of these and other high-sodium foods in your diet. High blood pressure medicine is usually more effective when such a diet is properly followed.

Also, it may be very important for you to go on a reducing diet. However, check with your doctor before changing your diet.

Many patients who have high blood pressure will not notice any signs of the problem. In fact, many may feel normal. It is very important that you **take your medicine exactly as directed** and that you keep your appointments with your doctor even if you feel well.

Remember that minoxidil will not cure your high blood pressure but it does help control it. Therefore, you must continue to take it as directed if you expect to lower your blood pressure and keep it down. **You may have to take high blood pressure medicine for the rest of your life.** If high blood pressure is not treated, it can cause serious problems such as heart failure, blood vessel disease, stroke, or kidney disease.

To help you remember to take your medicine, try to get into the habit of taking it at the same time each day.

This medicine is usually given together with certain other medicines. If you are using a combination of drugs, make sure that you take each medicine at the proper time and do not mix them. Ask your doctor, nurse, or pharmacist to help you plan a way to remember to take your medicines at the right time.

If you miss a dose of this medicine and remember it within a few hours, take it when you remember. However, if you do not remember until the next day, skip the missed dose and go back to your regular dosing schedule. Do not double doses.

How to store this medicine:

- **Keep out of the reach of children.**

- Store away from heat and direct light.

- Do not store in the bathroom, near the kitchen sink, or in other damp places. Heat or moisture may cause the medicine to break down.

- Do not keep outdated medicine or medicine no longer needed. Be sure that any discarded medicine is out of the reach of children.

Precautions While Using This Medicine

It is important that your doctor check your progress at regular visits to make sure that this medicine is working properly.

Ask your doctor about checking your pulse rate before and after taking minoxidil. Then, while you are taking this medicine, **check your pulse regularly while you are resting**. If it increases by 20 beats or more a minute, check with your doctor right away.

While you are taking minoxidil, **weigh yourself every day**. A weight gain of 2 to 3 pounds (about 1 kg) in an adult is normal and should be lost with continued treatment. However, if you suddenly gain 5 pounds (2 kg) or more (for a child, 2 pounds [1 kg] or more) or if you notice swelling of your feet or lower legs, check with your doctor right away.

Do not take other medicines unless they have been discussed with your doctor. This especially includes over-the-counter (nonprescription) medicines for appetite control, asthma, colds, cough, hay fever, or sinus problems, since they may tend to increase your blood pressure.

Side Effects of This Medicine

Along with its needed effects, a medicine may cause some unwanted effects. Although not all of these side effects may occur, if they do occur they may need medical attention.

Check with your doctor immediately if any of the following side effects occur:

More common

    Fast or irregular heartbeat
    Weight gain (rapid) of more than 5 pounds (2 pounds in children)

Less common

    Chest pains
    Shortness of breath

Check with your doctor as soon as possible if any of the following side effects occur:

More common
> Bloating
> Flushing or redness of skin
> Swelling of feet or lower legs

Less common
> Numbness or tingling of hands, feet, or face

Rare
> Skin rash and itching

Other side effects may occur that usually do not require medical attention. These side effects may go away during treatment as your body adjusts to the medicine. However, check with your doctor if any of the following side effects continue or are bothersome:

More common
> Increase in hair growth, usually on face, arms, and back

Less common or rare
> Breast tenderness in males and females
> Headache

This medicine causes a temporary increase in hair growth in most people. Hair may grow longer and darker in both men and women. This may first be noticed on the face several weeks after you start taking minoxidil. Later, new hair growth may be noticed on the back, arms, legs, and scalp. Talk to your doctor about shaving or using a hair remover during this time. After treatment with minoxidil has ended, the hair will stop growing, although it may take several months for the new hair growth to go away.

For elderly patients:

• Some medicines affect older patients differently than they do younger adults. Minoxidil may reduce tolerance to cold temperatures in elderly patients. Check with your doctor if this occurs. In addition, it is a good idea to check with your doctor or pharmacist if you notice any other unusual effects while taking this medicine or if you think it is not working as it should.

Other side effects not listed above may also occur in some patients. If you notice any other effects, check with your doctor.

PARGYLINE (Systemic)

A commonly used brand name in the U.S. is Eutonyl.

Pargyline (PAR-gi-leen) belongs to the group of medicines called antihypertensives. Specifically, it is a monoamine oxidase (MAO) inhibitor. It is taken by mouth to treat high blood pressure.

High blood pressure adds to the workload of the heart and arteries. If it continues for a long time, the heart and arteries may not function properly. This can damage the blood vessels of the brain, heart, and kidneys, resulting in a stroke, heart failure, or kidney failure. High blood pressure may also increase the risk of heart attacks. These problems may be less likely to occur if blood pressure is controlled.

Pargyline works by blocking the action of a chemical substance known as monoamine oxidase (MAO).

Pargyline is available only with your doctor's prescription.

Before Using This Medicine

To decide on the best treatment for your medical problem, your doctor should be told:

—if you have ever had any unusual or allergic reaction to pargyline.

—if you are on a low-salt, low-sugar, or any other special diet, or if you are allergic to any substance, such as foods, sulfites or other preservatives, or dyes. Most medicines contain more than their active ingredient. Your doctor, nurse, or pharmacist can help you avoid products that may cause a problem.

—if you are **pregnant** or if you may become pregnant. Studies have not been done in either humans or animals.

—if you are **breast-feeding**. Pargyline has not been shown to cause problems in nursing babies.

—if you have frequent headaches.

—if you have any of the following medical problems:
    Alcoholism (active)
    Angina (chest pain)
    Asthma or bronchitis
    Diabetes mellitus (sugar diabetes)

Epilepsy
Fever
Glaucoma
Headaches (severe or frequent)
Heart or blood vessel disease
Kidney disease
Liver disease
Mental illness (or history of)
Overactive thyroid
Parkinson's disease
Pheochromocytoma

—if you have recently had a heart attack or stroke.

—if you are now taking or have taken within the past 2 weeks any of the following medicines or types of medicine:

Carbamazepine (e.g., Tegretol)
Cyclobenzaprine (e.g., Flexeril)
Maprotiline (e.g., Ludiomil)
Other monoamine oxidase (MAO) inhibitors such as fura-
    zolidone (e.g., Furoxone), isocarboxazid (e.g., Marplan),
    phenelzine (e.g., Nardil), procarbazine (e.g., Matulane),
    or tranylcypromine (e.g., Parnate)
Tricyclic antidepressants (amitriptyline [e.g., Elavil], amox-
    apine [e.g., Asendin], clomipramine [e.g., Anafranil], de-
    sipramine [e.g., Pertofrane], doxepin [e.g., Sinequan],
    imipramine [e.g., Tofranil], nortriptyline [e.g., Aventyl],
    protriptyline [e.g., Vivactil], trimipramine [e.g., Surmon-
    til])

—if you are taking **any** other prescription or nonprescription (OTC) medicine, especially one that contains:

Amantadine (e.g., Symmetrel)
Amphetamines
Antidiabetics, oral (diabetes medicine you take by mouth)
Antidyskinetics (medicine for Parkinson's disease or other
    conditions affecting control of muscles)
Antihistamines
Antimuscarinics (medicine to help reduce stomach acid and
    for abdominal or stomach spasms or cramps)
Antipsychotics (medicine for mental illness)
Appetite suppressants (diet pills)
Buclizine (e.g., Bucladin)
Central nervous system (CNS) depressants
Chlophedianol (e.g., Ulo)
Cyclizine (e.g., Marezine)

Dextromethorphan (e.g., Delsym)
Disopyramide (e.g., Norpace)
Estrogens (female hormones)
Flavoxate (e.g., Urispas)
Fluoxetine (e.g., Prozac)
Guanadrel (e.g., Hylorel)
Guanethidine (e.g., Ismelin)
Insulin
Ipratropium (e.g., Atrovent)
Levodopa (e.g., Dopar)
Meclizine (e.g., Antivert)
Medicine for asthma or other breathing problems
Medicine for colds, sinus problems, or hay fever or other
    allergies (including nose drops or sprays)
Methyldopa (e.g., Aldomet)
Methylphenidate (e.g., Ritalin)
Orphenadrine (e.g., Norflex)
Oxybutinin (e.g., Ditropen)
Procainamide (e.g., Pronestyl)
Promethazine (e.g., Phenergan)
Quinidine (e.g., Quinidex)
Rauwolfia alkaloids (alseroxylon [e.g., Rauwiloid], deserpi-
    dine [e.g., Harmonyl], rauwolfia serpentina [e.g., Rau-
    dixin], reserpine [e.g., Serpasil])
Trimeprazine (e.g., Temaril)

—if you use cocaine. Cocaine use by individuals taking
pargyline or other MAO inhibitors may cause a severe
increase in blood pressure.

Proper Use of This Medicine

Importance of diet—When prescribing medicine for your
    condition, your doctor may also prescribe a personal diet
    for you. Such a diet may be low in sodium (salt). Most
    people eat much more sodium than they need and too
    much sodium in the diet may increase blood pressure.
    Some foods that contain large amounts of sodium are
    canned soup, pickles, ketchup, green and ripe olives, rel-
    ish, frankfurters, soy sauce, and carbonated beverages.
    Your doctor may want you to limit the amounts of these
    and other high-sodium foods in your diet. High blood
    pressure medicine is usually more effective when such a
    diet is properly followed.

Also, it may be very important for you to go on a reducing
    diet. However, check with your doctor before changing
    your diet.

Many patients who have high blood pressure will not notice any signs of the problem. In fact, many may feel normal. It is very important that you **take your medicine exactly as directed** and that you keep your appointments with your doctor even if you feel well.

Remember that this medicine will not cure your high blood pressure but it does help control it. Therefore, you must continue to take it as directed if you expect to lower your blood pressure and keep it down. **You may have to take high blood pressure medicine for the rest of your life.** If high blood pressure is not treated, it can cause serious problems such as heart failure, blood vessel disease, stroke, or kidney disease.

To help you remember to take your medicine, try to get into the habit of taking it at the same time each day.

If you miss a dose of this medicine and remember within 2 hours, take it right away and then go back to your regular dosing schedule. However, if you do not remember until later, skip the missed dose and go back to your regular dosing schedule. Do not double doses.

How to store this medicine:

- **Keep out of the reach of children.**

- Store away from heat and direct light.

- Do not store in the bathroom, near the kitchen sink, or in other damp places. Heat or moisture may cause the medicine to break down.

- Do not keep outdated medicine or medicine no longer needed. Be sure that any discarded medicine is out of the reach of children.

Precautions While Using This Medicine

It is important that your doctor check your progress at regular visits to make sure that this medicine is working properly and to check for unwanted effects.

Check with your doctor or hospital emergency room immediately if severe headache, stiff neck, chest pains, fast heartbeat, or nausea and vomiting occur while you are taking this medicine. These may be symptoms of a serious reaction which should have a doctor's attention.

When taken with certain foods, drinks, or other medicines, pargyline can cause very dangerous reactions such as sudden high blood pressure. To avoid such reactions, **obey the following rules of caution:**

• Do not eat foods that have a high tyramine content (most common in foods that are aged or fermented to increase their flavor), such as cheeses, yeast or meat extracts, fava or broad bean pods, smoked or pickled meat, poultry, or fish, fermented sausage (bologna, pepperoni, salami, and summer sausage) or other unfresh meat, or any overripe fruit. If a list of these foods and beverages is not given to you, ask your doctor, nurse, or pharmacist to provide one.

• Do not drink alcoholic beverages.

• Do not eat or drink large amounts of caffeine-containing food or beverages such as chocolate, coffee, tea, or cola.

• Do not take any other medicine unless approved or prescribed by your doctor. This especially includes over-the-counter (OTC) or nonprescription medicine such as that for colds (including nose drops), cough, asthma, hay fever, sinus problems, or appetite control; "keep awake" products; or products that make you sleepy.

After you stop using this medicine you must continue to obey the rules of caution concerning food, drink, and other medicine for at least 2 weeks. This medicine may continue to react with certain foods or other medicines for up to 14 days after you stop taking it.

This medicine will add to the effects of alcohol and other CNS depressants (medicines that slow down the nervous system, possibly causing drowsiness). Some examples of CNS depressants are antihistamines or medicine for hay fever, other allergies, or colds; sedatives, tranquilizers, or sleeping medicine; prescription pain medicine or narcotics; barbiturates; medicine for seizures; muscle relaxants; or anesthetics, including some dental anesthetics. **Check with your doctor before taking any of the above while you are using this medicine.**

This medicine may cause some people to become drowsy or less alert than they are normally. **Make sure you know how you react to this medicine before you drive, use machines, or do other jobs that could be dangerous if you are not alert.**

Dizziness, lightheadedness, or fainting may occur, especially when you get up from a lying or sitting position. **Getting up slowly may help.** When you get up from lying down, sit on the edge of the bed with your feet dangling for 1 or 2 minutes. Then stand up slowly. If the problem continues or gets worse, check with your doctor.

For diabetic patients:
• This medicine may affect blood sugar levels. While you are using this medicine, be especially careful in testing for sugar in your blood or urine. If you have any questions about this, check with your doctor.

Before having any kind of surgery (including dental surgery) or emergency treatment, tell the physician or dentist in charge that you are using this medicine or have used it within the past 2 weeks.

Your doctor may want you to carry an identification card stating that you are using this medicine.

Tell your doctor if you develop a fever since that may change the amount of medicine you have to take.

For patients with angina (chest pain):
• This medicine may cause you to have an unusual feeling of health and energy. However, **do not suddenly increase the amount of exercise you get without discussing it with your doctor.** To do so could bring on an attack of angina.

Side Effects of This Medicine

Along with its needed effects, a medicine may cause some unwanted effects. Although not all of these side effects may occur, if they do occur they may need medical attention.

Check with your doctor immediately if any of the following side effects occur:

Rare

 Chest pain (severe)
 Enlarged pupils
 Fast or slow heartbeat
 Headache (severe)
 Increased sensitivity of eyes to light
 Increased sweating (possibly with fever or cold, clammy skin)
 Nausea and vomiting
 Stiff or sore neck

Check with your doctor as soon as possible if any of the following side effects occur:

Less common

 Diarrhea
 Fainting
 Fast or pounding heartbeat
 Swelling of feet and lower legs

Rare

 Dark urine
 Hallucinations (seeing, hearing, or feeling things that are not there)
 Yellow eyes or skin

Other side effects may occur that usually do not require medical attention. These side effects may go away during treatment as your body adjusts to the medicine. However, check with your doctor if any of the following side effects continue or are bothersome:

More common

 Constipation
 Difficult urination
 Dizziness or lightheadedness, especially when getting up from a lying or sitting position
 Drowsiness
 Dry mouth
 Unusual tiredness and weakness

Less common or rare

 Increase in appetite and weight gain
 Increased sensitivity of skin to sunlight
 Muscle twitching during sleep
 Nightmares

Restlessness or agitation
Shakiness
Trouble in sleeping

For elderly patients:

• Some medicines affect older patients differently than they do younger adults. Dizziness, lightheadedness, or fainting, as well as other side effects, may be more likely to occur in the elderly, who are more sensitive to the effects of pargyline. Check with your doctor if these continue or are bothersome. In addition, it is a good idea to check with your doctor or pharmacist if you notice any other unusual effects while taking this medicine or if you think it is not working as it should.

Other side effects not listed above may also occur in some patients. If you notice any other effects, check with your doctor.

PARGYLINE AND METHYCLOTHIAZIDE
(Systemic)

A commonly used brand name in the U.S. is Eutron.

Pargyline (PAR-gi-leen) and methyclothiazide (meth-ee-kloe-THYE-a-zide) combination is taken by mouth to treat high blood pressure.

High blood pressure adds to the workload of the heart and arteries. If it continues for a long time, the heart and arteries may not function properly. This can damage the blood vessels of the brain, heart, and kidneys, resulting in a stroke, heart failure, or kidney failure. High blood pressure may also increase the risk of heart attacks. These problems may be less likely to occur if blood pressure is controlled.

Pargyline works by blocking the action of a chemical substance known as monoamine oxidase (MAO). The methyclothiazide in this combination is a thiazide diuretic (water pill) that helps reduce the amount of water in the body by increasing the flow of urine.

Pargyline and methyclothiazide combination is available only with your doctor's prescription.

Before Using This Medicine

To decide on the best treatment for your medical problem, your doctor should be told:

—if you have ever had any unusual or allergic reaction to pargyline, sulfonamides (sulfa drugs), indapamide, or methyclothiazide or any other thiazide diuretics (water pills).

—if you are on a low-salt, low-sugar, or any other special diet, or if you are allergic to any substance, such as foods, sulfites or other preservatives, or dyes. Most medicines contain more than their active ingredient. Your doctor, nurse, or pharmacist can help you avoid products that may cause a problem.

—if you are **pregnant** or if you may become pregnant. When methyclothiazide is used during pregnancy, it may cause side effects including jaundice, blood problems, and low potassium in the newborn infant. Studies with pargyline have not been done in either humans or animals.

—if you are **breast-feeding**. This medicine has not been shown to cause problems in nursing babies.

—if you have frequent headaches.

—if you have any of the following medical problems:
  Alcoholism (active)
  Angina (chest pain)
  Asthma or bronchitis
  Diabetes mellitus (sugar diabetes)
  Epilepsy
  Fever
  Glaucoma
  Gout (history of)
  Headaches (severe or frequent)
  Heart or blood vessel disease
  Kidney disease
  Liver disease
  Lupus erythematosus (or history of)
  Mental illness (history of)
  Overactive thyroid
  Pancreatitis (inflammation of the pancreas)
  Parkinson's disease
  Pheochromocytoma

—if you have recently had a heart attack or stroke.

—if you are now taking or have taken within the past 2 weeks any of the following medicines or types of medicine:
  Carbamazepine (e.g., Tegretol)
  Cyclobenzaprine (e.g., Flexeril)
  Maprotiline (e.g., Ludiomil)
  Other monoamine oxidase (MAO) inhibitors such as fura-zolidone (e.g., Furoxone), isocarboxazid (e.g., Marplan), phenelzine (e.g., Nardil), procarbazine (e.g., Matulane), or tranylcypromine (e.g., Parnate)
  Tricyclic antidepressants (amitriptyline [e.g., Elavil], amox-apine [e.g., Asendin], clomipramine [e.g., Anafranil], de-sipramine [e.g., Pertofrane], doxepin [e.g., Sinequan], imipramine [e.g., Tofranil], nortriptyline [e.g., Aventyl], protriptyline [e.g., Vivactil], trimipramine [e.g., Surmon-til])

—if you are taking **any** other prescription or nonprescription (OTC) medicine, especially one that contains:
  Adrenocorticoids (cortisone-like medicine)
  Amantadine (e.g., Symmetrel)

Antidiabetics, oral (diabetes medicine you take by mouth)
Antidyskinetics (medicine for Parkinson's disease or other
    conditions affecting control of muscles)
Antihistamines
Antimuscarinics (medicine to help reduce stomach acid and
    for abdominal or stomach spasms or cramps)
Antipsychotics (medicine for mental illness)
Buclizine (e.g., Bucladin)
Central nervous system (CNS) depressants
Chlophedianol (e.g., Ulo)
Cyclizine (e.g., Marezine)
Dextromethorphan (e.g., Delsym)
Digitalis glycosides (heart medicine)
Disopyramide (e.g., Norpace)
Estrogens (female hormones)
Flavoxate (e.g., Urispas)
Fluoxetine (e.g., Prozac)
Guanadrel (e.g., Hylorel)
Guanethidine (e.g., Ismelin)
Insulin
Ipratropium (e.g., Atrovent)
Levodopa (e.g., Dopar)
Lithium (e.g., Lithane)
Meclizine (e.g., Antivert)
Medicine for asthma or other breathing problems
Medicine for colds, sinus problems, or hay fever or other
    allergies (including nose drops or sprays)
Methenamine (e.g., Mandelamine)
Methyldopa (e.g., Aldomet)
Methylphenidate (e.g., Ritalin)
Orphenadrine (e.g., Norflex)
Oxybutinin (e.g., Ditropen)
Procainamide (e.g., Pronestyl)
Promethazine (e.g., Phenergan)
Quinidine (e.g., Quinidex)
Rauwolfia alkaloids (alseroxylon [e.g., Rauwiloid], deserpi-
    dine [e.g., Harmonyl], rauwolfia serpentina [e.g., Rau-
    dixin], reserpine [e.g., Serpasil])
Trimeprazine (e.g., Temaril)

—if you use cocaine. Cocaine use by individuals taking
pargyline (contained in this combination) or other MAO
inhibitors may cause a severe increase in blood pressure.

Proper Use of This Medicine

Importance of diet—When prescribing medicine for your
condition, your doctor may also prescribe a personal diet

for you. Such a diet may be low in sodium (salt). Most people eat much more sodium than they need and too much sodium in the diet may increase blood pressure. Some foods that contain large amounts of sodium are canned soup, pickles, ketchup, green and ripe olives, relish, frankfurters, soy sauce, and carbonated beverages. Your doctor may want you to limit the amounts of these and other high-sodium foods in your diet. High blood pressure medicine is usually more effective when such a diet is properly followed.

Also, it may be very important for you to go on a reducing diet. However, check with your doctor before changing your diet.

Many patients who have high blood pressure will not notice any signs of the problem. In fact, many may feel normal. It is very important that you **take your medicine exactly as directed** and that you keep your appointments with your doctor even if you feel well.

Remember that this medicine will not cure your high blood pressure but it does help control it. Therefore, you must continue to take it as directed if you expect to lower your blood pressure and keep it down. **You may have to take high blood pressure medicine for the rest of your life.** If high blood pressure is not treated, it can cause serious problems such as heart failure, blood vessel disease, stroke, or kidney disease.

This medicine may cause you to have an unusual feeling of tiredness when you begin to take it. You may also notice an increase in the amount of urine or in your frequency of urination. After taking the medicine for a while, these effects should lessen. To keep the increase in urine from affecting your nighttime sleep:

• If you are to take a single dose a day, take it in the morning after breakfast.

• If you are to take more than one dose a day, take the last dose no later than 6 p.m., unless otherwise directed by your doctor.

However, it is best to plan your dose or doses according to a schedule that will least affect your personal activities and sleep. Ask your doctor, nurse, or pharmacist to help you plan the best time to take this medicine.

To help you remember to take your medicine, try to get into the habit of taking it at the same time each day.

If you miss a dose of this medicine and remember within 2 hours, take it right away and then go back to your regular dosing schedule. If you do not remember until later, skip the missed dose and go back to your regular dosing schedule. Do not double doses.

How to store this medicine:

- **Keep out of the reach of children.**

- Store away from heat and direct light.

- Do not store in the bathroom, near the kitchen sink, or in other damp places. Heat or moisture may cause the medicine to break down.

- Do not keep outdated medicine or medicine no longer needed. Be sure that any discarded medicine is out of the reach of children.

Precautions While Using This Medicine

It is important that your doctor check your progress at regular visits to make sure that this medicine is working properly.

When taken with certain foods, drinks, or other medicines, pargyline and methyclothiazide combination can cause very dangerous reactions such as sudden high blood pressure. To avoid such reactions, **obey the following rules of caution:**

- Do not eat foods that have a high tyramine content (most common in foods that are aged or fermented to increase their flavor), such as cheeses, yeast or meat extracts, fava or broad bean pods, smoked or pickled meat, poultry, or fish, fermented sausage (bologna, pepperoni, salami, and summer sausage) or other unfresh meat, or any overripe fruit. If a list of these foods and beverages is not given to you, ask your doctor, nurse, or pharmacist to provide one.

- Do not drink alcoholic beverages.

- Do not eat or drink large amounts of caffeine-containing food or beverages such as chocolate, coffee, tea, or cola.

- Do not take any other medicine unless approved or prescribed by your doctor. This especially includes over-the-counter (OTC) or nonprescription medicine such as that for colds (including nose drops), cough, asthma, hay fever, sinus, or appetite control; "keep awake" products; or products that make you sleepy.

After you stop using this medicine you must continue to obey the rules of caution concerning food, drink, and other medicine for at least 2 weeks. This medicine may continue to react with certain foods or other medicines for up to 14 days after you stop taking it.

This medicine will add to the effects of alcohol and other CNS depressants (medicines that slow down the nervous system, possibly causing drowsiness). Some examples of CNS depressants are antihistamines or medicine for hay fever, other allergies, or colds; sedatives, tranquilizers, or sleeping medicine; prescription pain medicine or narcotics; barbiturates; medicine for seizures; muscle relaxants; or anesthetics, including some dental anesthetics. **Check with your doctor before taking any of the above while you are using this medicine.**

Before having any kind of surgery (including dental surgery) or emergency treatment, tell the physician or dentist in charge that you are using this medicine or have used it within the past 2 weeks.

This medicine may cause a loss of potassium from your body.

- To help prevent this, your doctor may want you to:

    —eat or drink foods that have a high potassium content (for example, orange or other citrus fruit juices), or

    —take a potassium supplement, or

    —take another medicine to help prevent the loss of the potassium in the first place.

• It is very important to follow these directions. Also, it is important not to change your diet on your own. This is more important if you are already on a special diet (as for diabetes), or if you are taking a potassium supplement or a medicine to reduce potassium loss. Extra potassium may not be necessary and, in some cases, too much potassium could be harmful.

For patients with angina (chest pain):

• This medicine may cause you to have an unusual feeling of health and energy. However, **do not suddenly increase the amount of exercise you get without discussing it with your doctor.** To do so could bring on an attack of angina.

For diabetic patients:

• This medicine may affect blood sugar levels. While you are using this medicine, be especially careful in testing for sugar in your blood or urine. If you have any questions about this, check with your doctor.

Your doctor may want you to carry an identification card stating that you are using this medicine.

Check with your doctor or hospital emergency room immediately if severe headache, stiff neck, chest pains, fast heartbeat, or nausea and vomiting occur while you are taking this medicine. These may be symptoms of a serious side reaction which should have a doctor's attention.

This medicine may cause some people to become drowsy or less alert than they are normally. **Make sure you know how you react to this medicine before you drive, use machines, or do other jobs that could be dangerous if you are not alert.**

Dizziness, lightheadedness, or fainting may occur, especially when you get up from a lying or sitting position. **Getting up slowly may help.** When you get up from lying down, sit on the edge of the bed with your feet dangling for 1 or 2 minutes. Then stand up slowly. If the problem continues or gets worse, check with your doctor.

Tell your doctor if you develop a fever since that may change the amount of medicine you have to take.

Check with your doctor if you become sick and have severe
or continuing vomiting or diarrhea. These problems may
cause you to lose additional water and potassium.

Some people who take this medicine may become more sensitive to sunlight than they are normally. **When you first
begin taking this medicine, avoid too much sun and do not
use a sunlamp until you see how you react to the sun,
especially if you tend to burn easily. If you have a severe
reaction, check with your doctor.**

Side Effects of This Medicine

Along with its needed effects, a medicine may cause some
unwanted effects. Although not all of these side effects
may occur, if they do occur they may need medical attention.

Check with your doctor immediately if any of the following
side effects occur:

Rare

    Chest pain (severe)
    Enlarged pupils
    Fast or slow heartbeat
    Headache (severe)
    Increased sensitivity of eyes to light
    Increased sweating (possibly with fever or cold, clammy skin)
    Nausea and vomiting
    Stiff or sore neck

Check with your doctor as soon as possible if any of the
following side effects occur:

Less common

    Fainting
    Fast or pounding heartbeat
    Swelling of feet and lower legs

Rare

    Dark urine
    Fever
    Hallucinations (seeing, hearing, or feeling things that are not
        there)
    Joint, lower back or side, or stomach pain
    Skin rash or hives
    Sore throat and fever

Stomach pain (severe) with nausea and vomiting
Unusual bleeding or bruising
Yellow eyes or skin

Signs and symptoms of too much potassium loss

Dryness of mouth
Increased thirst
Irregular heartbeats
Mood or mental changes
Muscle cramps or pain
Nausea or vomiting
Unusual tiredness or weakness
Weak pulse

Other side effects may occur that usually do not require medical attention. These side effects may go away during treatment as your body adjusts to the medicine. However, check with your doctor if any of the following side effects continue or are bothersome:

More common

Constipation
Difficult urination
Dizziness or lightheadedness, especially when getting up from a lying or sitting position
Drowsiness

Less common or rare

Decreased sexual ability
Increased sensitivity of skin to sunlight
Insomnia
Muscle twitching during sleep
Nightmares
Restlessness or agitation
Shakiness

For elderly patients:

• Some medicines may affect older patients differently than they do younger adults. Dizziness, lightheadedness, or fainting, symptoms of too much potassium loss, as well as other side effects, may be more likely to occur in the elderly, who are usually more sensitive to the effects of this medicine. Check with your doctor if these occur. In addition, it is a good idea to check with your doctor or pharmacist if you notice any other unusual effects while taking this medicine or if you think it is not working as it should.

Other side effects not listed above may also occur in some patients. If you notice any other effects, check with your doctor.

PHENOXYBENZAMINE (Systemic)

A commonly used brand name in the U.S. is Dibenzyline.

Phenoxybenzamine (fen-ox-ee-BEN-za-meen) belongs to the general class of medicines called antihypertensives. It is taken by mouth to treat high blood pressure due to a disease called pheochromocytoma. It is also used to treat some problems due to poor blood circulation.

Phenoxybenzamine blocks the effects of certain chemicals in the body. When these chemicals are present in large amounts, they cause high blood pressure.

Phenoxybenzamine is available only with your doctor's prescription.

Before Using This Medicine

To decide on the best treatment for your medical problem, your doctor should be told:

—if you have ever had any unusual or allergic reaction to phenoxybenzamine.

—if you are on a low-salt, low-sugar, or any other special diet, or if you are allergic to any substance, such as foods, sulfites or other preservatives, or dyes. Most medicines contain more than their active ingredient. Your doctor, nurse, or pharmacist can help you avoid products that may cause a problem.

—if you are **pregnant** or if you may become pregnant. Studies have not been done in either humans or animals.

—if you are **breast-feeding**. However, phenoxybenzamine has not been shown to cause problems in nursing babies.

—if you have any of the following medical problems:

    Angina (chest pain)
    Heart or blood vessel disease
    Kidney disease
    Lung infection

—if you have recently had a heart attack or stroke.

—if you are taking **any** other prescription or nonprescription (OTC) medicine.

Proper Use of This Medicine

In order to help remember to take your medicine, try to get into the habit of taking it at the same time each day.

If you miss a dose of this medicine, take it as soon as you remember. However, if it is almost time for your next dose, skip the missed dose and go back to your regular dosing schedule. Do not double doses.

How to store this medicine:

• **Keep out of the reach of children.**

• Store away from heat and direct light.

• Do not store in the bathroom, near the kitchen sink, or in other damp places. Heat or moisture may cause the medicine to break down.

• Do not keep outdated medicine or medicine no longer needed. Be sure that any discarded medicine is out of the reach of children.

Precautions While Using This Medicine

It is important that your doctor check your progress at regular visits to make sure that this medicine is working properly and to check for unwanted effects.

Do not take other medicines unless they have been discussed with your doctor. This especially includes over-the-counter (nonprescription) medicines for appetite control, asthma, colds, cough, hay fever, or sinus problems, since they may interfere with the effects of this medicine.

Phenoxybenzamine may cause some people to become dizzy, drowsy, or less alert than they are normally. This is more likely to happen when you begin to take it or when you increase the amount of medicine you are taking. **Make sure you know how you react to this medicine before you drive, use machines, or do other jobs that could be dangerous if you are not alert.**

Dizziness, lightheadedness, or fainting may occur, especially when you get up from a lying or sitting position. Getting

up slowly may help, but if the problem continues or gets worse, check with your doctor.

The dizziness, lightheadedness, or fainting is also more likely to occur if you drink alcohol, stand for a long time, exercise, or if the weather is hot. **While you are taking this medicine, be careful in the amount of alcohol you drink. Also, use extra care during exercise or hot weather or if you must stand for a long time.**

Before having any kind of surgery (including dental surgery) or emergency treatment, **tell the physician or dentist in charge that you are using this medicine.**

Phenoxybenzamine may cause dryness of the mouth, nose, and throat. For temporary relief of mouth dryness, use sugarless candy or gum, melt bits of ice in your mouth, or use a saliva substitute. However, if dry mouth continues for more than 2 weeks, check with your physician or dentist. Continuing dryness of the mouth may increase the chance of dental disease, including tooth decay, gum disease, and fungus infections.

Side Effects of This Medicine

In rats and mice, phenoxybenzamine has been found to increase the risk of development of malignant tumors. It is not known if phenoxybenzamine increases the chance of tumors in humans.

Along with its needed effects, a medicine may cause some unwanted effects. The following side effects may go away as your body adjusts to the medicine. However, check with your doctor if any of these effects continue or are bothersome:

More common
> Dizziness or lightheadedness, especially when getting up from a lying or sitting position
> Fast heartbeat
> Pinpoint pupils
> Stuffy nose

Less common
> Confusion
> Drowsiness

Dry mouth
Headache
Lack of energy
Sexual problems in males
Unusual tiredness or weakness

For elderly patients:

• Some medicines may affect older patients differently than they do younger adults. Dizziness or light-headedness may be more likely to occur in the elderly, who are more sensitive to the effects of phenoxybenzamine. In addition, phenoxybenzamine may reduce tolerance to cold temperatures in elderly patients. Check with your doctor if these occur. In addition, it is a good idea to check with your doctor or pharmacist if you notice any other unusual effects while taking this medicine or if you think it is not working as it should.

Other side effects not listed above may also occur in some patients. If you notice any other effects, check with your doctor.

PRAZOSIN (Systemic)

A commonly used brand name in the U.S. and Canada is Minipress.

Prazosin (PRA-zoe-sin) belongs to the general class of medicines called antihypertensives. It is taken by mouth to treat high blood pressure.

High blood pressure adds to the workload of the heart and arteries. If it continues for a long time, the heart and arteries may not function properly. This can damage the blood vessels of the brain, heart, and kidneys, resulting in a stroke, heart failure, or kidney failure. High blood pressure may also increase the risk of heart attacks. These problems may be less likely to occur if blood pressure is controlled.

Prazosin works by relaxing blood vessels so that blood passes through them more easily. This helps to lower blood pressure.

Prazosin may also be used for other conditions as determined by your doctor.

Prazosin is available only with your doctor's prescription.

Before Using This Medicine

To decide on the best treatment for your medical problem, your doctor should be told:

—if you have ever had any unusual or allergic reaction to prazosin.

—if you are on a low-salt, low-sugar, or any other special diet, or if you are allergic to any substance, such as foods, sulfites or other preservatives, or dyes. Most medicines contain more than their active ingredient. Your doctor, nurse, or pharmacist can help you avoid products that may cause a problem.

—if you are **pregnant** or if you may become pregnant Studies have not been done in humans. However, prazosin has not been shown to cause birth defects or other problems in animals.

—if you are **breast-feeding**. However, prazosin has not been shown to cause problems in nursing babies.

—if you have any of the following medical problems:
   Angina (chest pain)
   Heart disease
   Kidney disease

—if you are taking any other prescription or nonprescription (OTC) medicine.

Proper Use of This Medicine

Importance of diet—When prescribing medicine for your condition, your doctor may also prescribe a personal diet for you. Such a diet may be low in sodium (salt). Most people eat much more sodium than they need and too much sodium in the diet may increase blood pressure. Some foods that contain large amounts of sodium are canned soup, pickles, ketchup, green and ripe olives, relish, frankfurters, soy sauce, and carbonated beverages. Your doctor may want you to limit the amounts of these and other high-sodium foods in your diet. High blood pressure medicine is usually more effective when such a diet is properly followed.

Also, it may be very important for you to go on a reducing diet. However, check with your doctor before changing your diet.

Many patients who have high blood pressure will not notice any signs of the problem. In fact, many may feel normal. It is very important that you **take your medicine exactly as directed** and that you keep your appointments with your doctor even if you feel well.

Remember that prazosin will not cure your high blood pressure but it does help control it. Therefore, you must continue to take it as directed if you expect to lower your blood pressure and keep it down. **You may have to take high blood pressure medicine for the rest of your life.** If high blood pressure is not treated, it can cause serious problems such as heart failure, blood vessel disease, stroke, or kidney disease.

To help you remember to take your medicine, try to get into the habit of taking it at the same time each day.

If you miss a dose of this medicine, take it as soon as possible. However, if it is almost time for your next dose, skip the missed dose and go back to your regular dosing schedule. Do not double doses.

How to store this medicine:
- **Keep out of the reach of children.**
- Store away from heat and direct light.
- Do not store in the bathroom, near the kitchen sink, or in other damp places. Heat or moisture may cause the medicine to break down.
- Do not keep outdated medicine or medicine no longer needed. Be sure that any discarded medicine is out of the reach of children.

Precautions While Using This Medicine

It is important that your doctor check your progress at regular visits to make sure that this medicine is working properly.

Do not take other medicines unless they have been discussed with your doctor. This especially includes over-the-counter (nonprescription) medicines for appetite control, asthma, colds, cough, hay fever, or sinus problems, since they may tend to increase your blood pressure.

Dizziness and irregular heartbeat may occur after the first dose of this medicine. Taking the first dose at bedtime may prevent problems. However, **be especially careful if you need to get up during the night.** Make sure you know how you react to this medicine before you drive, use machines, or do other jobs that could be dangerous if you are not alert. After you have taken several doses of this medicine, these effects should lessen.

Dizziness, lightheadedness, or fainting may occur, especially when you get up from a lying or sitting position. Getting up slowly may help lessen this problem. **If you begin to feel dizzy, lie down so that you do not faint.** Then sit for a few moments before standing to prevent the dizziness from returning.

The dizziness, lightheadedness, or fainting is also more likely to occur if you drink alcohol, stand for a long time, exercise, or if the weather is hot. **While you are taking this medicine, be careful in the amount of alcohol you drink. Also, use extra care during exercise or hot weather or if you must stand for a long time.**

Side Effects of This Medicine

Along with its needed effects, a medicine may cause some unwanted effects. Although not all of these side effects may occur, if they do occur they may need medical attention.

Check with your doctor as soon as possible if any of the following side effects occur:

Less common

Chest pain
Dizziness or lightheadedness, especially when getting up from a lying or sitting position
Fainting (sudden)
Irregular heartbeat
Shortness of breath
Swelling of feet or lower legs
Weight gain

Rare

Inability to control urination
Numbness or tingling of hands or feet

Other side effects may occur that usually do not require medical attention. These side effects may go away during treatment as your body adjusts to the medicine. However, check with your doctor if any of the following side effects continue or are bothersome:

Less common

Drowsiness
Headache
Lack of energy
Nausea and vomiting

For elderly patients:

• Some medicines may affect older patients differently than they do younger adults. Dizziness, lightheadedness, or fainting may be more likely to occur in the elderly, who are more sensitive to the effects of prazosin. In addition, prazosin may reduce tolerance to cold temperatures in elderly patients. Check with your doctor if this occurs. In addition, it is a good idea to check with your doctor or pharmacist if you notice any other unusual effects while taking this medicine or if you think it is not working as it should.

Other side effects not listed above may also occur in some patients. If you notice any other effects, check with your doctor.

PRAZOSIN AND POLYTHIAZIDE
(Systemic)†

A commonly used brand name in the U.S. is Minizide.

†Not commercially available in Canada.

Prazosin (PRA-zoe-sin) and polythiazide (pol-i-THYE-a-zide) combination is used in the treatment of high blood pressure.

High blood pressure adds to the workload of the heart and arteries. If it continues for a long time, the heart and arteries may not function properly. This can damage the blood vessels of the brain, heart, and kidneys resulting in a stroke, heart failure, or kidney failure. High blood pressure may also increase the risk of heart attacks. These problems may be less likely to occur if blood pressure is controlled.

Prazosin works by relaxing blood vessels so that blood passes through them more easily. The polythiazide in this combination is a thiazide diuretic (water pill) that helps to reduce the amount of water in the body by increasing the flow of urine. Both of these actions help to lower blood pressure.

This medicine is available only with your doctor's prescription.

Before Using This Medicine

To decide on the best treatment for your medical problem, your doctor should be told:

—if you have ever had any unusual or allergic reaction to prazosin, sulfonamides (sulfa drugs), or any of the thiazide diuretics.

—if you are on a low-salt, low-sugar, or any other special diet, or if you are allergic to any substance, such as foods, sulfites or other preservatives, or dyes. Most medicines contain more than their active ingredient. Your doctor, nurse, or pharmacist can help you avoid products that may cause a problem.

—if you are **pregnant** or if you may become pregnant. When polythiazide (contained in this combination medicine) is used during pregnancy, it may cause side effects including jaundice, blood problems, and low potassium in the newborn infant. The combination of prazosin and polythiazide has not been shown to cause birth defects.

—if you are **breast-feeding**. Polythiazide passes into breast milk. However, prazosin and polythiazide combination has not been shown to cause problems in nursing babies.

—if you have any of the following medical problems:

Angina (chest pain)
Diabetes mellitus (sugar diabetes)
Gout (history of)
Heart disease
Kidney disease
Liver disease
Lupus erythematosus (history of)
Pancreatitis (inflammation of the pancreas)

—if you are taking **any** other prescription or nonprescription (OTC) medicine, especially one that contains:

Adrenocorticoids (cortisone-like medicines)
Digitalis glycosides (heart medicine)
Lithium (e.g., Lithane)
Methenamine (e.g., Mandelamine)

Proper Use of This Medicine

Importance of diet—When prescribing medicine for your condition, your doctor may also prescribe a personal diet for you. Such a diet may be low in sodium (salt). Most people eat much more sodium than they need and too much sodium in the diet may increase blood pressure. Some foods that contain large amounts of sodium are canned soup, pickles, ketchup, green and ripe olives, relish, frankfurters, soy sauce, and carbonated beverages. Your doctor may want you to limit the amounts of these and other high-sodium foods in your diet. High blood pressure medicine is usually more effective when such a diet is properly followed.

Also, it may be very important for you to go on a reducing diet. However, check with your doctor before changing your diet.

Many patients who have high blood pressure will not notice any signs of the problem. In fact, many may feel normal.

It is very important that you **take your medicine exactly as directed** and that you keep your appointments with your doctor even if you feel well.

Remember that this medicine will not cure your high blood pressure but it does help control it. Therefore, you must continue to take it as directed if you expect to lower your blood pressure and keep it down. **You may have to take high blood pressure medicine for the rest of your life.** If high blood pressure is not treated, it can cause serious problems such as heart failure, blood vessel disease, stroke, or kidney disease.

This medicine may cause you to have an unusual feeling of tiredness when you begin to take it. You may also notice an increase in the amount of urine or in your frequency of urination. After taking the medicine for a while, these effects should lessen. To keep the increase in urine from affecting your nighttime sleep:

• If you are to take a single dose a day, take it in the morning after breakfast.

• If you are to take more than one dose a day, take the last dose no later than 6 p.m., unless otherwise directed by your doctor.

However, it is best to plan your dose or doses according to a schedule that will least affect your personal activities and sleep. Ask your doctor, nurse, or pharmacist to help you plan the best time to take this medicine.

To help you remember to take your medicine, try to get into the habit of taking it at the same time each day.

If you miss a dose of this medicine, take it as soon as possible. However, if it is almost time for your next dose, skip the missed dose and go back to your regular dosing schedule. Do not double doses.

How to store this medicine:

• **Keep out of the reach of children.**

• Store away from heat and direct light.

• Do not store in the bathroom, near the kitchen sink, or

in other damp places. Heat or moisture may cause the medicine to break down.

• Do not keep outdated medicine or medicine no longer needed. Be sure that any discarded medicine is out of the reach of children.

Precautions While Using This Medicine

It is important that your doctor check your progress at regular visits to make sure this medicine is working properly.

Do not take other medicines unless they have been discussed with your doctor. This especially includes over-the-counter (nonprescription) medicine for appetite control, asthma, colds, cough, hay fever, or sinus problems, since they may tend to increase your blood pressure.

This medicine may cause a loss of potassium from your body.

• To help prevent this, your doctor may want you to:

—eat or drink foods that have a high potassium content (for example, orange or other citrus fruit juices), or

—take a potassium supplement, or

—take another medicine to help prevent the loss of the potassium in the first place.

• It is very important to follow these directions. Also, it is important not to change your diet on your own. This is more important if you are already on a special diet (as for diabetes), or if you are taking a potassium supplement or a medicine to reduce potassium loss. Extra potassium may not be necessary and, in some cases, too much potassium could be harmful.

Check with your doctor if you become sick and have severe or continuing vomiting or diarrhea. These problems may cause you to lose additional water and potassium.

Dizziness and irregular heartbeat may occur after the first dose of this medicine. Taking the first dose at bedtime may prevent problems. However, **be especially careful if you need to get up during the night.** Also, **avoid driving** or performing hazardous tasks for the first 24 hours after you start taking this medicine or when the dose is increased. **Make sure you know how you react to this medicine before you drive, use machines, or do other jobs that could be dangerous if you are not alert.** After you have taken several doses of this medicine, these effects should lessen.

Dizziness, lightheadedness, or fainting may occur, especially when you get up from a lying or sitting position. Getting up slowly may help lessen this problem. **If you begin to feel dizzy, lie down so that you do not faint.** Then sit for a few moments before standing to prevent the dizziness from returning.

The dizziness, lightheadedness, or fainting is also more likely to occur if you drink alcohol, stand for a long time, exercise, or if the weather is hot. **While you are taking this medicine, be careful in the amount of alcohol you drink. Also, use extra care during exercise or hot weather or if you must stand for a long time.**

For diabetic patients:

• Polythiazide (contained in this combination medicine) may raise blood sugar levels. While you are using this medicine, be especially careful in testing for sugar in your blood or urine. If you have any questions about this, check with your doctor.

Some people who take this medicine may become more sensitive to sunlight than they are normally. When you first begin taking this medicine, avoid too much sun and do not use a sunlamp until you see how you react to the sun, especially if you tend to burn easily. If you have a severe reaction, check with your doctor.

Side Effects of This Medicine

Along with its needed effects, a medicine may cause some unwanted effects. Although not all of these side effects may occur, if they do occur they may need medical attention.

Check with your doctor as soon as possible if any of the
following side effects occur, especially since some of them
may mean that your body is losing too much potassium:

Signs and symptoms of too much potassium loss

Dryness of mouth (severe)
Increased thirst
Irregular heartbeat (continuing)
Mood or mental changes
Muscle cramps or pain
Nausea or vomiting
Unusual tiredness or weakness
Weak pulse

More common

Dizziness or lightheadedness, especially when getting up from
a lying or sitting position

Less common

Chest pain
Fainting (sudden)
Irregular heartbeat
Shortness of breath
Swelling of feet or lower legs
Weight gain

Rare

Inability to control urination
Joint, lower back or side, or stomach pain
Numbness or tingling of hands or feet
Skin rash or hives
Sore throat and fever
Stomach pain (severe) with nausea and vomiting
Unusual bleeding or bruising
Yellow eyes or skin

Other side effects may occur that usually do not require
medical attention. These side effects may go away
during treatment as your body adjusts to the medicine.
However, check with your doctor if any of the following side effects continue or are bothersome:

Less common

Decreased sexual ability
Diarrhea
Drowsiness
Headache
Increased sensitivity of skin to sunlight

Lack of energy
Loss of appetite
Stomach upset or pain

For elderly patients:

• Some medicines may affect older patients differently than they do younger adults. Dizziness, lightheadedness, or fainting or symptoms of too much potassium loss may be more likely to occur in the elderly, who are more sensitive to the effects of prazosin and polythiazide. In addition, this medicine may reduce tolerance to cold temperatures in elderly patients. Check with your doctor if this occurs. In addition, it is a good idea to check with your doctor or pharmacist if you notice any other unusual effects while taking this medicine or if you think it is not working as it should.

Other side effects not listed above may also occur in some patients. If you notice any other effects, check with your doctor.

RAUWOLFIA ALKALOIDS (Systemic)

This information applies to the following medicines:

    Alseroxylon (al-ser-OX-i-lon)
    Deserpidine (de-SER-pi-deen)
    Rauwolfia Serpentina (rah-WOOL-fee-a ser-pen-TEE-na)
    Reserpine (re-SER-peen)

Some commonly used brand names are:

For Alseroxylon†
In the U.S.
    Rauwiloid

For Deserpidine†
In the U.S.
    Harmonyl

For Rauwolfia Serpentina†
In the U.S.

Raudixin	Rauverid
Rauval	Wolfina

    Generic name product may also be available.

For Reserpine
In the U.S.
    Serpalan
    Serpasil

    Generic name product may also be available.

In Canada

Novoreserpine	Serpasil
Reserfia	

    Generic name product may also be available.

---

    †Not commercially available in Canada.

Rauwolfia alkaloids belong to the general class of medicines called antihypertensives. They are taken by mouth to treat high blood pressure.

High blood pressure adds to the workload of the heart and arteries. If it continues for a long time, the heart and arteries may not function properly. This can damage the blood vessels of the brain, heart, and kidneys, resulting in a stroke, heart failure, or kidney failure. High blood pressure may also increase the risk of heart attacks. These problems may be less likely to occur if blood pressure is controlled.

Rauwolfia alkaloids work by controlling nerve impulses along certain nerve pathways. As a result, they act on the heart and blood vessels to lower blood pressure.

Rauwolfia alkaloids may also be used to treat other conditions as determined by your doctor.

These medicines are available only with your doctor's prescription.

Before Using This Medicine

To decide on the best treatment for your medical problem, your doctor should be told:

—if you have ever had any unusual or allergic reaction to rauwolfia alkaloids.

—if you are on a low-salt, low-sugar, or any other special diet, or if you are allergic to any substance, such as foods, sulfites or other preservatives, or dyes. Most medicines contain more than their active ingredient. Your doctor, nurse, or pharmacist can help you avoid products that may cause a problem.

—if you are **pregnant** or if you may become pregnant. Too much use of rauwolfia alkaloids during pregnancy may cause unwanted effects (difficult breathing, low temperature, loss of appetite) in the baby. In rats, use of rauwolfia alkaloids during pregnancy causes birth defects and in guinea pigs decreases newborn survival rates. Be sure you have discussed this with your doctor before taking this medicine.

—if you are **breast-feeding**. Rauwolfia alkaloids pass into the breast milk and may cause unwanted effects (difficult breathing, low temperature, loss of appetite) in infants of mothers taking large doses of this medicine. Be sure you have discussed this with your doctor before taking this medicine.

—if you have any of the following medical problems:
Allergies or other breathing problems such as asthma
Epilepsy
Gallstones
Heart disease
Kidney disease
Mental depression (or history of)
Parkinson's disease
Pheochromocytoma
Stomach ulcer
Ulcerative colitis

—if you are now taking or have taken within the past 2 weeks monoamine oxidase (MAO) inhibitors, such as:

Furazolidone (e.g., Furoxone)
Isocarboxazid (e.g., Marplan)
Pargyline (e.g., Eutonyl)
Phenelzine (e.g., Nardil)
Procarbazine (e.g., Matulane)
Tranylcypromine (e.g., Parnate)

—if you are taking **any** other prescription or nonprescription (OTC) medicine.

Proper Use of This Medicine

For patients taking this medicine for high blood pressure:

• Importance of diet—When prescribing medicine for your condition, your doctor may also prescribe a personal diet for you. Such a diet may be low in sodium (salt). Most people eat much more sodium than they need and too much sodium in the diet may increase blood pressure. Some foods that contain large amounts of sodium are canned soup, pickles, ketchup, green and ripe olives, relish, frankfurters, soy sauce, and carbonated beverages. Your doctor may want you to limit the amounts of these and other high-sodium foods in your diet. High blood pressure medicine is usually more effective when such a diet is properly followed.

Also, it may be very important for you to go on a reducing diet. However, check with your doctor before changing your diet.

• Many patients who have high blood pressure will not notice any signs of the problem. In fact, many may feel normal. It is very important that you **take your medicine exactly as directed** and that you keep your appointments with your doctor even if you feel well.

• Remember that this medicine will not cure your high blood pressure but it does help control it. Therefore, you must continue to take it as directed if you expect to lower your blood pressure and keep it down. **You may have to take high blood pressure medicine for the rest of your life.** If high blood pressure is not treated, it can cause serious

problems such as heart failure, blood vessel disease, stroke, or kidney disease.

To help you remember to take your medicine, try to get into the habit of taking it at the same time each day.

This medicine is sometimes given together with certain other medicines. If you are using a combination of drugs, make sure that you take each medicine at the proper time and do not mix them. Ask your doctor, nurse, or pharmacist to help you plan a way to remember to take your medicines at the right times.

If this medicine upsets your stomach, it may be taken with meals or milk. If stomach upset (nausea, vomiting, stomach cramps or pain) continues or gets worse, check with your doctor.

If you miss a dose of this medicine, do not take the missed dose at all and do not double the next one. Instead, go back to your regular dosing schedule.

How to store this medicine:

• **Keep out of the reach of children.**

• Store away from heat and direct light.

• Do not store in the bathroom, near the kitchen sink, or in other damp places. Heat or moisture may cause the medicine to break down.

• Do not keep outdated medicine or medicine no longer needed. Be sure that any discarded medicine is out of the reach of children.

Precautions While Using This Medicine

It is important that your doctor check your progress at regular visits to make sure that this medicine is working properly.

For patients taking this medicine for high blood pressure:

• **Do not take other medicines unless they have been discussed with your doctor.** This especially includes over-the-counter (nonprescription) medicines for appetite control, asthma, colds, cough, hay fever, or sinus problems, since they may tend to increase your blood pressure.

Before having any kind of surgery (including dental surgery) or emergency treatment, **tell the physician or dentist in charge that you are taking this medicine.**

In some patients, this medicine may cause mental depression. **Tell your doctor right away:**

—if you or anyone else notices unusual changes in your mood.

—if you start having early-morning sleeplessness or unusually vivid dreams or nightmares.

This medicine will add to the effects of alcohol and other CNS depressants (medicines that slow down the nervous system, possibly causing drowsiness). Some examples of CNS depressants are antihistamines or medicine for hay fever, other allergies, or colds; sedatives, tranquilizers, or sleeping medicine; prescription pain medicine or narcotics; barbiturates; medicine for seizures; muscle relaxants; or anesthetics, including some dental anesthetics. **Check with your doctor before taking any of the above while you are using this medicine.**

This medicine may cause some people to become drowsy or less alert than they are normally. This is more likely to happen when you begin to take it or when you increase the amount of medicine you are taking. **Make sure you know how you react to this medicine before you drive, use machines, or do other jobs that could be dangerous if you are not alert.**

This medicine may cause dryness of the mouth. For temporary relief, use sugarless candy or gum, melt bits of ice in your mouth, or use a saliva substitute. However, if dry mouth continues for more than 2 weeks, check with your physician or dentist. Continuing dryness of the mouth may increase the chance of dental disease, including tooth decay, gum disease, and fungus infections.

This medicine often causes stuffiness in the nose. However, do not use nasal decongestant medicines without first checking with your doctor or pharmacist.

Side Effects of This Medicine

Suggestions that rauwolfia alkaloids may increase the risk of breast cancer occurring later have not been proven. However, rats and mice given 100 to 300 times the human dose had an increased number of tumors.

Along with its needed effects, a medicine may cause some unwanted effects. Although not all of these side effects may occur, if they do occur they may need medical attention.

Check with your doctor immediately if any of the following side effects occur:

Less common

Drowsiness or faintness
Impotence or decreased sexual interest
Lack of energy or weakness
Mental depression or inability to concentrate
Nervousness or anxiety
Vivid dreams or nightmares or early-morning sleeplessness

Check with your doctor as soon as possible if any of the following side effects occur:

More common

Dizziness

Less common

Black tarry stools
Bloody vomit
Chest pain
Headache
Irregular or slow heartbeat
Shortness of breath
Stomach cramps or pain

Rare

Painful or difficult urination
Skin rash or itching
Stiffness
Trembling and shaking of hands and fingers
Unusual bleeding or bruising

Signs and symptoms of overdose

Dizziness or drowsiness (severe)
Flushing of skin

Pinpoint pupils of eyes
Slow pulse

Other side effects may occur that usually do not require medical attention. These side effects may go away during treatment as your body adjusts to the medicine. However, check with your doctor if any of the following side effects continue or are bothersome:

More common
Diarrhea
Dry mouth
Loss of appetite
Nausea and vomiting
Stuffy nose

Less common
Swelling of feet and lower legs

For elderly patients:

• Some medicines may affect older patients differently than they do younger adults. Dizziness may be more likely to occur in the elderly, who are more sensitive to the effects of rauwolfia alkaloids. Check with your doctor if this occurs. In addition, it is a good idea to check with your doctor or pharmacist if you notice any other unusual effects while taking this medicine or if you think it is not working as it should.

After you stop using this medicine, it may still produce some side effects that need attention. During this period of time **check with your doctor immediately** if you notice any of the following side effects:

Drowsiness or faintness
Impotence or decreased sexual interest
Irregular or slow heartbeat
Lack of energy or weakness
Mental depression or inability to concentrate
Nervousness or anxiety
Vivid dreams or nightmares or early-morning sleeplessness

Other side effects not listed above may also occur in some patients. If you notice any other effects, check with your doctor.

RAUWOLFIA ALKALOIDS AND THIAZIDE DIURETICS
(Systemic)

This information applies to the following medicines:

Deserpidine (de-SER-pi-deen) and Hydrochlorothiazide (hye-droe-klor-oh-THYE-a-zide)

Deserpidine and Methyclothiazide (meth-i-kloe-THYE-a-zide)

Rauwolfia Serpentina (rah-WOOL-fee-a ser-pen-TEE-na) and Bendroflumethiazide (ben-droe-floo-meth-EYE-a-zide)

Reserpine (re-SER-peen) and Chlorothiazide (klor-oh-THYE-a-zide)

Reserpine and Chlorthalidone (klor-THAL-i-done)

Reserpine and Hydrochlorothiazide

Reserpine and Hydroflumethiazide (hye-droe-floo-meth-EYE-a-zide)

Reserpine and Methyclothiazide

Reserpine and Polythiazide (pol-i-THYE-a-zide)

Reserpine and Quinethazone (kwin-ETH-a-zone)

Reserpine and Trichlormethiazide (trye-klor-meth-EYE-a-zide)

Some commonly used brand names are:

For Deserpidine and Hydrochlorothiazide†
In the U.S.
        Oreticyl
        Oreticyl Forte

For Deserpidine and Methyclothiazide
In the U.S.
        Enduronyl
        Enduronyl Forte

     Generic name product may also be available.

In Canada
        Dureticyl

For Rauwolfia Serpentina and Bendroflumethiazide†
In the U.S.
        Rauzide

For Reserpine and Chlorothiazide†
In the U.S.
        Diupres
        Diurigen with Reserpine

     Generic name product may also be available.

For Reserpine and Chlorthalidone†
In the U.S.
        Demi-Regroton
        Regroton

For Reserpine and Hydrochlorothiazide
In the U.S.

Hydropres	Mallopres
Hydrosine	Serpasil-Esidrix
Hydrotensin	

Generic name product may also be available.

In Canada
   Hydropres
   Serpasil-Esidrix

For Reserpine and Hydroflumethiazide
In the U.S.

Hydropine	Salutensin
Hydropine H.P.	Salutensin-Demi
Salazide	

Generic name product may also be available.

In Canada
   Salutensin

For Reserpine and Methyclothiazide†
In the U.S.
   Diutensen-R

For Reserpine and Polythiazide†
In the U.S.
   Renese-R

For Reserpine and Quinethazone†
In the U.S.
   Hydromox R

For Reserpine and Trichlormethiazide†
In the U.S.

Diurese-R	Naquival
Metatensin	

Generic name product may also be available.

---

†Not commercially available in Canada.

Rauwolfia alkaloid and thiazide diuretic combinations are used in the treatment of high blood pressure.

High blood pressure adds to the workload of the heart and arteries. If it continues for a long time, the heart and arteries may not function properly. This can damage the blood vessels of the brain, heart, and kidneys, resulting in a stroke, heart failure, or kidney failure. High blood pressure may also increase the risk of heart attacks. These problems may be less likely to occur if blood pressure is controlled.

Rauwolfia alkaloids work by controlling nerve impulses along certain nerve pathways. As a result, they act on the heart and blood vessels to lower blood pressure. Thiazide diuretics help to reduce the amount of water in the body by increasing the flow of urine. This also helps to lower blood pressure.

These medicines are available only with your doctor's prescription.

Before Using This Medicine

To decide on the best treatment for your medical problem, your doctor should be told:

—if you have ever had any unusual or allergic reaction to sulfonamides (sulfa drugs), thiazide diuretics (water pills), or rauwolfia alkaloids.

—if you are on a low-salt, low-sugar, or any other special diet, or if you are allergic to any substance, such as foods, sulfites or other preservatives, or dyes. Most medicines contain more than their active ingredient. Your doctor, nurse, or pharmacist can help you avoid products that may cause a problem.

—if you are **pregnant** or if you may become pregnant. Too much use of thiazide diuretics (contained in this combination medicine) during pregnancy may cause unwanted effects including jaundice, blood problems, and low potassium in the baby. Too much use of rauwolfia alkaloids may cause difficult breathing, low temperature, and loss of appetite in the baby. This medicine has not been shown to cause birth defects in humans. In rats, use of rauwolfia alkaloids during pregnancy decreases newborn survival rates. Be sure that you have discussed this with your doctor before taking this medicine.

—if you are **breast-feeding**. Rauwolfia alkaloids pass into the breast milk and may cause unwanted effects (difficult breathing, low temperature, loss of appetite) in infants of mothers taking large doses of it. Be sure you have discussed this with your doctor before taking this medicine.

—if you have any of the following medical problems:
Allergies or other breathing problems such as asthma
Diabetes mellitus (sugar diabetes)
Epilepsy
Gallstones

  Gout (history of)
  Heart disease
  Kidney disease
  Liver disease
  Lupus erythematosus (history of)
  Mental depression (or history of)
  Pancreatitis (inflammation of pancreas)
  Parkinson's disease
  Pheochromocytoma
  Stomach ulcer
  Ulcerative colitis

—if you are now taking or have taken within the past 2 weeks monoamine oxidase (MAO) inhibitors such as:

  Furazolidone (e.g., Furoxone)
  Isocarboxazid (e.g., Marplan)
  Pargyline (e.g., Eutonyl)
  Phenelzine (e.g., Nardil)
  Procarbazine (e.g., Matulane)
  Tranylcypromine (e.g., Parnate)

—if you are taking **any** other prescription or nonprescription (OTC) medicine, especially one that contains:

  Adrenocorticoids (cortisone-like medicines)
  Digitalis glycosides (heart medicine)
  Lithium (e.g., Lithane)
  Methenamine (e.g., Mandelamine)

Proper Use of This Medicine

Importance of diet—When prescribing medicine for your condition, your doctor may also prescribe a personal diet for you. Such a diet may be low in sodium (salt). Most people eat much more sodium than they need and too much sodium in the diet may increase blood pressure. Some foods that contain large amounts of sodium are canned soup, pickles, ketchup, green and ripe olives, relish, frankfurters, soy sauce, and carbonated beverages. Your doctor may want you to limit the amounts of these and other high-sodium foods in your diet. High blood pressure medicine is usually more effective when such a diet is properly followed.

Also, it may be very important for you to go on a reducing diet. However, check with your doctor before changing your diet.

Many patients who have high blood pressure will not notice any signs of the problem. In fact, many may feel normal. It is very important that you **take your medicine exactly as directed** and that you keep your appointments with your doctor even if you feel well.

Remember that this medicine will not cure your high blood pressure but it does help control it. Therefore, you must continue to take it as directed if you expect to lower your blood pressure and keep it down. **You may have to take high blood pressure medicine for the rest of your life.** If high blood pressure is not treated, it can cause serious problems such as heart failure, blood vessel disease, stroke, or kidney disease.

This medicine may cause you to have an unusual feeling of tiredness when you begin to take it. You may also notice an increase in the amount of urine or in your frequency of urination. After you have taken the medicine for a while, these effects should lessen. In general, to keep the increase in urine from affecting your sleep:

• If you are to take a single dose a day, take it in the morning after breakfast.

• If you are to take more than one dose a day, take the last dose no later than 6 p.m., unless otherwise directed by your doctor.

However, it is best to plan your dose or doses according to a schedule that will least affect your personal activities and sleep. Ask your doctor, nurse, or pharmacist to help you plan the best time to take this medicine.

To help you remember to take your medicine, try to get into the habit of taking it at the same time each day.

If this medicine upsets your stomach, it may be taken with meals or milk. If stomach upset (nausea, vomiting, stomach pain or cramps) continues, check with your doctor.

If you miss a dose of this medicine, take it as soon as possible. However, if it is almost time for your next dose, skip the missed dose and go back to your regular dosing schedule. Do not double doses.

How to store this medicine:

- **Keep out of the reach of children.**

- Store away from heat and direct light.

- Do not store in the bathroom, near the kitchen sink, or in other damp places. Heat or moisture may cause the medicine to break down.

- Do not keep outdated medicine or medicine no longer needed. Be sure that any discarded medicine is out of the reach of children.

Precautions While Using This Medicine

It is important that your doctor check your progress at regular visits to make sure that this medicine is working properly.

Do not take other medicines unless they have been discussed with your doctor. This especially includes over-the-counter (nonprescription) medicines for appetite control, asthma, colds, cough, hay fever, or sinus problems, since they may tend to increase your blood pressure.

Before having any kind of surgery (including dental surgery), or emergency treatment, **tell the physician or dentist in charge that you are taking this medicine.**

This medicine may cause a loss of potassium from your body.

- To help prevent this, your doctor may want you to:

    —eat or drink foods that have a high potassium content (for example, orange or other citrus fruit juices), or

    —take a potassium supplement, or

    —take another medicine to help prevent the loss of the potassium in the first place.

- It is very important to follow these directions. Also, it is important not to change your diet on your own. This is more important if you are already on a special diet (as for diabetes), or if you are taking a potassium supplement or a medicine to reduce potassium loss. Extra potassium may not be necessary and, in some cases, too much potassium could be harmful.

Check with your doctor if you become sick and have severe or continuing vomiting or diarrhea. These problems may cause you to lose additional water and potassium.

This medicine may cause some people to become drowsy or less alert than they are normally. This is more likely to happen when you begin to take it or when you increase the amount of medicine you are taking. **Make sure you know how you react to this medicine before you drive, use machines, or do other jobs that could be dangerous if you are not alert.**

Dizziness, lightheadedness, or fainting may occur, especially when you get up from a lying or sitting position. Getting up slowly may help but if the problem continues or gets worse, check with your doctor.

In some patients, this medicine may cause mental depression. **Tell your doctor right away:**

—if you or anyone else notices unusual changes in your moods.

—if you start having early-morning sleeplessness or unusually vivid dreams or nightmares.

This medicine will add to the effects of alcohol and other CNS depressants (medicines that slow down the nervous system, possibly causing drowsiness). Some examples of CNS depressants are antihistamines or medicine for hay fever, other allergies, or colds; sedatives, tranquilizers, or sleeping medicine; prescription pain medicine or narcotics; barbiturates; medicine for seizures; muscle relaxants; or anesthetics, including dental anesthetics. **Check with your doctor before taking any of the above while you are taking this medicine.**

For diabetic patients:

• This medicine may raise blood sugar levels. While you are using this medicine, be especially careful in testing for sugar in your urine. If you have any questions about this, check with your doctor.

A few people who take this medicine may become more sensitive to sunlight than they are normally. When you first begin taking this medicine, avoid too much sun and do not use a sunlamp until you see how you react to the sun, especially if you tend to burn easily. If you have a severe reaction, check with your doctor.

This medicine often causes stuffiness in the nose. However, do not use nasal decongestant medicines without first checking with your doctor or pharmacist.

This medicine may cause dryness of the mouth. For temporary relief, use sugarless candy or gum, melt bits of ice in your mouth, or use a saliva substitute. However, if dry mouth continues for more than 2 weeks, check with your physician or dentist. Continuing dryness of the mouth may increase the chance of dental disease, including tooth decay, gum disease, and fungus infections.

Side Effects of This Medicine

Suggestions that rauwolfia alkaloids may increase the risk of breast cancer occurring later have not been proven. However, rats and mice given 100 to 300 times the human dose had an increased risk of tumors.

Along with its needed effects, a medicine may cause some unwanted effects. Although not all of these side effects may occur, if they do occur they may need medical attention.

Check with your doctor immediately if any of the following side effects occur:

Less common
> Drowsiness or faintness
> Impotence or decreased sexual interest
> Lack of energy or weakness
> Mental depression or inability to concentrate
> Nervousness or anxiety
> Vivid dreams or nightmares or early-morning sleeplessness

Check with your doctor as soon as possible if any of the following side effects occur:

Less common
> Black tarry stools
> Bloody vomit

Chest pain
Headache
Irregular or slow heartbeat
Joint pain
Shortness of breath

Rare

Painful or difficult urination
Skin rash or itching
Sore throat and fever
Stiffness
Stomach pain (severe) with nausea and vomiting
Trembling and shaking of hands and fingers
Unusual bleeding or bruising
Yellow eyes or skin

Symptoms of too much potassium loss or overdose

Dry mouth
Increased thirst
Muscle cramps or pain
Nausea or vomiting

Other signs and symptoms of overdose

Dizziness or drowsiness, severe
Flushing of skin
Pinpoint pupils of eyes
Slow pulse

Other side effects may occur that usually do not require medical attention. These side effects may go away during treatment as your body adjusts to the medicine. However, check with your doctor if any of the following side effects continue or are bothersome:

More common

Diarrhea
Dizziness, especially when getting up from a lying or sitting position
Loss of appetite
Stuffy nose

For elderly patients:

• Some medicines may affect older patients differently than they do younger adults. Dizziness or faintness or symptoms of too much potassium loss may be more likely to occur in the elderly, who are more sensitive to the effects of rauwolfia alkaloids and thiazide diuretics. Check with your doctor if these occur. In addition, it is a good idea to check with your doctor or pharmacist if you notice any other unusual effects while taking this medicine or if you think it is not working as it should.

After you stop using this medicine, it may still produce some side effects that need attention. During this period of time **check with your doctor immediately** if you notice any of the following side effects:

    Drowsiness or faintness
    Impotence or decreased sexual interest
    Irregular or slow heartbeat
    Lack of energy or weakness
    Mental depression or inability to concentrate
    Nervousness or anxiety
    Vivid dreams or nightmares or early-morning sleeplessness

Other side effects not listed above may also occur in some patients. If you notice any other effects, check with your doctor.

RESERPINE AND HYDRALAZINE
(Systemic)†

A commonly used brand name in the U.S. is Serpasil-Apresoline.

†Not commercially available in Canada.

The reserpine (re-SER-peen) and hydralazine (hye-DRAL-a-zeen) combination is taken by mouth to treat high blood pressure.

High blood pressure adds to the workload of the heart and arteries. If it continues for a long time, the heart and arteries may not function properly. This can damage the blood vessels of the brain, heart, and kidneys, resulting in a stroke, heart failure, or kidney failure. High blood pressure may also increase the risk of heart attacks. These problems may be less likely to occur if blood pressure is controlled.

Reserpine works by controlling nerve impulses along certain nerve pathways. As a result, it acts on the heart and blood vessels to lower blood pressure. Hydralazine works by relaxing blood vessels and increasing the supply of blood and oxygen to the heart while reducing its work load.

Reserpine and hydralazine combination is available only with your doctor's prescription.

Before Using This Medicine

To decide on the best treatment for your medical problem, your doctor should be told:

—if you have ever had any unusual or allergic reaction to rauwolfia alkaloids or hydralazine.

—if you are on a low-salt, low-sugar, or any other special diet, or if you are allergic to any substance, such as foods, sulfites or other preservatives, or dyes. Most medicines contain more than their active ingredient. Your doctor, nurse, or pharmacist can help you avoid products that may cause a problem.

—if you are **pregnant** or if you may become pregnant. Too much use of reserpine during pregnancy may cause unwanted effects (difficult breathing, low temperature, loss of appetite) in the baby. In rats, rauwolfia alkaloids decrease the newborn survival rate. Studies in mice have shown that hydralazine causes birth defects (cleft palate, defects in head and face bones); these birth defects may also occur in rabbits, but do not occur in rats; studies have not been done in humans. Be sure that you have discussed this with your doctor before taking this medicine.

—if you are **breast-feeding**. Reserpine passes into the breast milk and may cause unwanted effects (difficult breathing, low temperature, loss of appetite) in infants of mothers taking large doses of it. Hydralazine has not been shown to cause problems in nursing babies. Be sure you have discussed this with your doctor before taking this medicine.

—if you have recently had a stroke.

—if you have any of the following medical problems:
Allergies or other breathing problems, such as asthma
Epilepsy
Gallstones
Heart disease
Kidney disease
Mental depression (or history of)
Parkinson's disease
Pheochromocytoma (PCC)
Stomach ulcer
Ulcerative colitis

—if you are now taking or have taken within the past 2 weeks monoamine oxidase (MAO) inhibitors, such as:
Furazolidone (e.g., Furoxone)
Isocarboxazid (e.g., Marplan)
Pargyline (e.g., Eutonyl)
Phenelzine (e.g., Nardil)
Procarbazine (e.g., Matulane)
Tranylcypromine (e.g., Parnate)

—if you are taking **any** other prescription or nonprescription (OTC) medicine.

Proper Use of This Medicine

Importance of diet—When prescribing medicine for your condition, your doctor may also prescribe a personal diet for you. Such a diet may be low in sodium (salt). Most people eat much more sodium than they need and too much sodium in the diet may increase blood pressure. Some foods that contain large amounts of sodium are canned soup, pickles, ketchup, green and ripe olives, relish, frankfurters, soy sauce, and carbonated beverages. Your doctor may want you to limit the amounts of these and other high-sodium foods in your diet. High blood pressure medicine is usually more effective when such a diet is properly followed.

Also, it may be very important for you to go on a reducing diet. However, check with your doctor before changing your diet.

Many patients who have high blood pressure will not notice any signs of the problem. In fact, many may feel normal. It is very important that you **take your medicine exactly as directed** and that you keep your appointments with your doctor even if you feel well.

Remember that this medicine will not cure your high blood pressure but it does help control it. Therefore, you must continue to take it as directed if you expect to lower your blood pressure and keep it down. **You may have to take high blood pressure medicine for the rest of your life.** If high blood pressure is not treated, it can cause serious problems such as heart failure, blood vessel disease, stroke, or kidney disease.

To help you remember to take your medicine, try to get into the habit of taking it at the same time each day.

If this medicine upsets your stomach, it may be taken with meals or milk. If stomach upset (nausea, vomiting, stomach pain, or cramps) continues, check with your doctor.

If you miss a dose of this medicine, take it as soon as possible. However, if it is almost time for your next dose, skip the missed dose and go back to your regular dosing schedule. Do not double doses.

How to store this medicine:
- **Keep out of the reach of children.**
- Store away from heat and direct light.

• Do not store in the bathroom, near the kitchen sink, or in other damp places. Heat or moisture may cause the medicine to break down.

• Do not keep outdated medicine or medicine no longer needed. Be sure that any discarded medicine is out of the reach of children.

Precautions While Using This Medicine

It is important that your doctor check your progress at regular visits to make sure that this medicine is working properly.

Do not take other medicines unless they have been discussed with your doctor. This especially includes over-the-counter (nonprescription) medicine for appetite control, asthma, colds, cough, hay fever, or sinus problems, since they may tend to increase your blood pressure.

Before having any kind of surgery (including dental surgery), or emergency treatment, **make sure the physician or dentist in charge knows that you are taking this medicine.**

This medicine may cause some people to have headaches or to feel dizzy or drowsy. **Make sure you know how you react to this medicine before you drive, use machines, or do other jobs that could be dangerous if you are not alert.**

In some patients, this medicine may cause mental depression. **Tell your doctor right away:**

—if you or anyone else notices unusual changes in your mood.

—if you start having early-morning sleeplessness or unusually vivid dreams or nightmares.

This medicine will add to the effects of alcohol and other CNS depressants (medicines that slow down the nervous system, possibly causing drowsiness). Some examples of CNS depressants are antihistamines or medicine for hay fever, other allergies, or cold; sedatives, tranquilizers, or sleeping medicine; prescription pain medicine or narcotics; barbiturates; medicine for seizures; muscle relaxants; or anesthetics, including dental anesthetics. **Check with**

your doctor before taking any of the above while you are taking this medicine.

This medicine often causes stuffiness in the nose. However, do not use nasal decongestant medicines without first checking with your doctor or pharmacist.

This medicine may cause dryness of the mouth. For temporary relief, use sugarless candy or gum, melt bits of ice in your mouth, or use a saliva substitute. However, if dry mouth continues for more than 2 weeks, check with your physician or dentist. Continuing dryness of the mouth may increase the chance of dental disease, including tooth decay, gum disease, and fungus infections.

Side Effects of This Medicine

Suggestions that rauwolfia alkaloids (like reserpine) may increase the risk of breast cancer occurring later have not been proven. However, rats and mice given 100 to 300 times the human dose had an increased number of tumors.

Along with its needed effects, a medicine may cause some unwanted effects. Although not all of these side effects may occur, if they do occur they may need medical attention.

Check with your doctor immediately if any of the following side effects occur:

More common

General feeling of body discomfort or weakness

Less common

Drowsiness or faintness
Impotence or decreased sexual interest
Mental depression or inability to concentrate
Nervousness or anxiety
Vivid dreams or nightmares or early-morning sleeplessness

Check with your doctor as soon as possible if any of the following side effects occur:

Less common

Black tarry stools
Blisters on skin

Bloody vomit
Chest pain
Fever and sore throat
Headache
Irregular heartbeat
Joint pain
Numbness, tingling, pain, or weakness in hands or feet
Shortness of breath
Skin rash or itching
Swelling of feet or lower legs
Swelling of lymph glands

Rare

Painful or difficult urination
Stiffness
Stomach pain (severe) with nausea and vomiting
Trembling and shaking of hands and fingers
Unusual bleeding or bruising

Signs and symptoms of overdose

Dizziness or drowsiness (severe)
Flushing of skin
Pinpoint pupils of eyes
Slow pulse

Other side effects may occur that usually do not require medical attention. These side effects may go away during treatment as your body adjusts to the medicine. However, check with your doctor if any of the following side effects continue or are bothersome:

More common

Diarrhea
Dizziness
Dry mouth
Loss of appetite
Nausea or vomiting
Stuffy nose

Less common

Constipation
Flushing or redness of skin
Red, sore eyes

For elderly patients:

• Some medicines may affect older patients differently than they do younger adults. Dizziness or faintness may be more likely to occur in the elderly, who are more sensitive to the effects of reserpine and hydralazine. Also, this medicine may reduce tolerance to cold temperatures in elderly patients. Check with your doctor if these occur. In addition, it is a good idea to check with your doctor or pharmacist if you notice any other unusual effects while taking this medicine or if you think it is not working as it should.

After you stop using this medicine, it may still produce some side effects that need attention. During this period of time **check with your doctor immediately** if you notice any of the following side effects:

    Drowsiness or faintness
    General feeling of body discomfort or weakness
    Impotence or decreased sexual interest
    Irregular or slow heartbeat
    Mental depression or inability to concentrate
    Nervousness or anxiety
    Vivid dreams or nightmares or early-morning sleeplessness

Other side effects not listed above may also occur in some patients. If you notice any other effects, check with your doctor.

RESERPINE, HYDRALAZINE, AND HYDROCHLOROTHIAZIDE (Systemic)

Some commonly used brand names are:

In the U.S.

Cam-Ap-Es	Ser-Ap-Es
Cherapas	Serpazide
Ser-A-Gen	Tri-Hydroserpine
Seralazide	Unipres

Generic name product may also be available.

In Canada

Ser-Ap-Es

Reserpine (re-SER-peen), hydralazine (hye-DRAL-a-zeen), and hydrochlorothiazide (hye-droe-KLOR-oh-THYE-a-zide) combinations are taken by mouth to treat high blood pressure.

High blood pressure adds to the workload of the heart and arteries. If it continues for a long time, the heart and arteries may not function properly. This can damage the blood vessels of the brain, heart, and kidneys, resulting in a stroke, heart failure, or kidney failure. High blood pressure may also increase the risk of heart attacks. These problems may be less likely to occur if blood pressure is controlled.

Reserpine works by controlling nerve impulses along certain nerve pathways. As a result, it acts on the heart and blood vessels to lower blood pressure. Hydralazine works by relaxing blood vessels and increasing the supply of blood to the heart while reducing its work load. Hydrochlorothiazide is a thiazide diuretic (water pill) that helps to reduce the amount of water in the body by increasing the flow of urine. This also helps to lower blood pressure.

This medicine is available only with your doctor's prescription.

Before Using This Medicine

To decide on the best treatment for your medical problem, your doctor should be told:

—if you have ever had any unusual or allergic reaction to hydralazine, sulfonamides (sulfa drugs), thiazide diuretics (water pills), or rauwolfia alkaloids.

—if you are on a low-salt, low-sugar, or any other special diet, or if you are allergic to any substance, such as foods, sulfites or other preservatives, or dyes. Most medicines contain more than their active ingredient. Your doctor, nurse, or pharmacist can help you avoid products that may cause a problem.

—if you are **pregnant** or if you may become pregnant. Too much use of reserpine and hydrochlorothiazide during pregnancy may cause unwanted effects (jaundice, blood problems, low potassium, difficult breathing, low temperatures, and loss of appetite) in the baby. In rats, rauwolfia alkaloids (like reserpine) decrease newborn survival rates. Studies in mice have shown that hydralazine causes birth defects (cleft palate, defects in head and face bones); these birth defects may also occur in rabbits, but do not occur in rats; studies have not been done in humans. Be sure that you have discussed this with your doctor before taking this medicine.

—if you are **breast-feeding**. Reserpine passes into the breast milk and may cause unwanted effects (difficult breathing, low temperature, loss of appetite) in infants of mothers taking large doses of it. Hydrochlorothiazide also passes into breast milk. Be sure you have discussed this with your doctor before taking this medicine.

—if you have any of the following medical problems:
Allergies or other breathing problems such as asthma
Diabetes mellitus (sugar diabetes)
Epilepsy
Gallstones
Gout (history of)
Heart disease
Kidney disease
Liver disease
Lupus erythematosus (history of)
Mental depression (or history of)
Pancreatitis (inflammation of pancreas)
Parkinson's disease
Pheochromocytoma
Stomach ulcer
Ulcerative colitis

—if you have recently had a stroke.

—if you are now taking or have taken within the past 2 weeks monoamine oxidase (MAO) inhibitors, such as:

Furazolidone (e.g., Furoxone)
Isocarboxazid (e.g., Marplan)
Pargyline (e.g., Eutonyl)
Phenelzine (e.g., Nardil)
Procarbazine (e.g., Matulane)
Tranylcypromine (e.g., Parnate)

—if you are taking **any** other prescription or nonprescription (OTC) medicine, especially one that contains:

Adrenocorticoids (cortisone-like medicines)
Digitalis glycosides (heart medicine)
Lithium (e.g., Lithane)
Methenamine (e.g., Mandelamine)

Proper Use of This Medicine

Importance of diet—When prescribing medicine for your condition, your doctor may also prescribe a personal diet for you. Such a diet may be low in sodium (salt). Most people eat much more sodium than they need and too much sodium in the diet may increase blood pressure. Some foods that contain large amounts of sodium are canned soup, pickles, ketchup, green and ripe olives, relish, frankfurters, soy sauce, and carbonated beverages. Your doctor may want you to limit the amounts of these and other high-sodium foods in your diet. High blood pressure medicine is usually more effective when such a diet is properly followed.

Also, it may be very important for you to go on a reducing diet. However, check with your doctor before changing your diet.

Many patients who have high blood pressure will not notice any signs of the problem. In fact, many may feel normal. It is very important that you **take your medicine exactly as directed** and that you keep your appointments with your doctor even if you feel well.

Remember that this medicine will not cure your high blood pressure but it does help control it. Therefore, you must continue to take it as directed if you expect to lower your blood pressure and keep it down. **You may have to take**

high blood pressure medicine for the rest of your life. If high blood pressure is not treated, it can cause serious problems such as heart failure, blood vessel disease, stroke, or kidney disease.

This medicine may cause you to have an unusual feeling of tiredness when you begin to take it. You may also notice an increase in the amount of urine or in your frequency of urination. After you have taken the medicine for a while, these effects should lessen. In general, to keep the increase in urine from affecting your sleep:

• If you are to take a single dose a day, take it in the morning after breakfast.

• If you are to take more than one dose a day, take the last dose no later than 6 p.m., unless otherwise directed by your doctor.

However, it is best to plan your dose or doses according to a schedule that will least affect your personal activities and sleep. Ask your doctor, nurse, or pharmacist to help you plan the best time to take this medicine.

To help you remember to take your medicine, try to get into the habit of taking it at the same time each day.

If this medicine upsets your stomach, it may be taken with meals or milk. If stomach upset (nausea, vomiting, stomach pain or cramps) continues, check with your doctor.

If you miss a dose of this medicine, take it as soon as possible. However, if it is almost time for your next dose, skip the missed dose and go back to your regular dosing schedule. Do not double doses.

How to store this medicine:

• **Keep out of the reach of children.**

• Store away from heat and direct light.

• Do not store in the bathroom, near the kitchen sink, or in other damp places. Heat or moisture may cause the medicine to break down.

• Do not keep outdated medicine or medicine no longer needed. Be sure that any discarded medicine is out of the reach of children.

Precautions While Using This Medicine

It is important that your doctor check your progress at regular visits to make sure that this medicine is working properly.

Do not take other medicines unless they have been discussed with your doctor. This especially includes over-the-counter (nonprescription) medicines for appetite control, asthma, colds, cough, hay fever, or sinus problems, since they may tend to increase your blood pressure.

Before having any kind of surgery (including dental surgery), or emergency treatment, **make sure the physician or dentist in charge knows that you are taking this medicine.**

This medicine may cause some people to have headaches or to feel dizzy or drowsy. **Make sure you know how you react to this medicine before you drive, use machines, or do other jobs that could be dangerous if you are not alert.**

Dizziness, lightheadedness, or fainting may occur, especially when you get up from a lying or sitting position. Getting up slowly may help, but if the problem continues or gets worse, check with your doctor.

In some patients, this medicine may cause mental depression. **Tell your doctor right away:**

—if you or anyone else notices unusual changes in your mood.

—if you start having early-morning sleeplessness or unusually vivid dreams or nightmares.

This medicine will add to the effects of alcohol and other CNS depressants (medicines that slow down the nervous system, possibly causing drowsiness). Some examples of CNS depressants are antihistamines or medicine for hay fever, other allergies, or colds; sedatives, tranquilizers, or sleeping medicine; prescription pain medicine or narcotics; barbiturates; medicine for seizures; muscle relaxants; or anesthetics, including dental anesthetics. **Check with your doctor before taking any of the above while you are taking this medicine.**

This medicine may cause a loss of potassium from your body.

- To help prevent this, your doctor may want you to:

  —eat or drink foods that have a high potassium content (for example, orange or other citrus fruit juices), or

  —take a potassium supplement, or

  —take another medicine to help prevent the loss of the potassium in the first place.

- It is very important to follow these directions. Also, it is important not to change your diet on your own. This is more important if you are already on a special diet (as for diabetes), or if you are taking a potassium supplement or a medicine to reduce potassium loss. Extra potassium may not be necessary and, in some cases, too much potassium could be harmful.

For diabetic patients:

- This medicine may raise blood sugar levels. While you are using this medicine, be especially careful in testing for sugar in your urine. If you have any questions about this, check with your doctor.

A few people who take this medicine may become more sensitive to sunlight than they are normally. When you first begin taking this medicine, avoid too much sun and do not use a sunlamp until you see how you react to the sun, especially if you tend to burn easily. If you have a severe reaction, check with your doctor.

This medicine often causes stuffiness in the nose. However, do not use nasal decongestant medicines without first checking with your doctor or pharmacist.

This medicine may cause dryness of the mouth. For temporary relief, use sugarless candy or gum, melt bits of ice in your mouth, or use a saliva substitute. However, if dry mouth continues for more than 2 weeks, check with your physician or dentist. Continuing dryness of the mouth may increase the chance of dental disease, including tooth decay, gum disease, and fungus infections.

Side Effects of This Medicine

Suggestions that rauwolfia alkaloids may increase the risk of breast cancer occurring later have not been proven. However, rats and mice given 100 to 300 times the human dose had an increased number of tumors.

Along with its needed effects, a medicine may cause some unwanted effects. Although not all of these side effects may occur, if they do occur they may need medical attention.

Check with your doctor immediately if any of the following side effects occur:

More common

General feeling of body discomfort or weakness

Less common

Drowsiness or faintness
Impotence or decreased sexual interest
Mental depression or inability to concentrate
Nervousness or anxiety
Vivid dreams or nightmares or early-morning sleeplessness

Check with your doctor as soon as possible if any of the following side effects occur:

Less common

Black tarry stools
Blisters on skin
Bloody vomit
Chest pain
Fever and sore throat
Headache
Irregular heartbeat
Joint pain
Numbness, tingling, pain, or weakness in hands or feet
Shortness of breath
Skin rash or itching
Swelling of lymph glands

Rare

Painful or difficult urination
Stiffness
Stomach pain (severe) with nausea and vomiting
Trembling and shaking of hands and fingers

Unusual bleeding or bruising
Yellow eyes or skin

Signs and symptoms of overdose
Dizziness or drowsiness (severe)
Dryness of mouth
Flushing of skin
Increased thirst
Muscle cramps or pain
Nausea or vomiting (severe)
Pinpoint pupils of eyes
Slow pulse

Other side effects may occur that usually do not require medical attention. These side effects may go away during treatment as your body adjusts to the medicine. However, check with your doctor if any of the following side effects continue or are bothersome:

More common
Diarrhea
Dizziness, especially when getting up from a lying or sitting position
Loss of appetite
Nausea or vomiting
Stuffy nose

Less common
Constipation
Flushing or redness of skin
Red, sore eyes

For elderly patients:

• Some medicines may affect older patients differently than they do younger adults. Dizziness or faintness or symptoms of too much potassium loss may be more likely to occur in the elderly, who are more sensitive to the effects of this medicine. Also, this medicine may reduce tolerance to cold temperatures in elderly patients. Check with your doctor if these occur. In addition, it is a good idea to check with your doctor or pharmacist if you notice any other unusual effects while taking this medicine or if you think it is not working as it should.

After you stop using this medicine, it may still produce
some side effects that need attention. During this period of time **check with your doctor immediately** if you
notice any of the following side effects:

Drowsiness or faintness
General feeling of body discomfort or weakness
Impotence or decreased sexual interest
Irregular heartbeat
Mental depression or inability to concentrate
Nervousness or anxiety
Vivid dreams or nightmares or early-morning sleeplessness

Other side effects not listed above may also occur in some
patients. If you notice any other effects, check with your
doctor.

TERAZOSIN (Systemic)†

A commonly used brand name in the U.S. is Hytrin.

---

†Not commercially available in Canada.

Terazosin (ter-AY-zoe-sin) belongs to the general class of medicines called antihypertensives. It is taken by mouth to treat high blood pressure.

High blood pressure adds to the workload of the heart and arteries. If it continues for a long time, the heart and arteries may not function properly. This can damage the blood vessels of the brain, heart, and kidneys, resulting in a stroke, heart failure, or kidney failure. High blood pressure may also increase the risk of heart attacks. These problems may be less likely to occur if blood pressure is controlled.

Terazosin works by relaxing blood vessels so that blood passes through them more easily. This helps to lower blood pressure.

Terazosin is available only with your doctor's prescription.

Before Using This Medicine

To decide on the best treatment for your medical problem, your doctor should be told:

—if you have ever had any unusual or allergic reaction to terazosin.

—if you are on a low-salt, low-sugar, or any other special diet, or if you are allergic to any substance, such as foods, sulfites or other preservatives, or dyes. Most medicines contain more than their active ingredient. Your doctor, nurse, or pharmacist can help you avoid products that may cause a problem.

—if you are **pregnant** or if you may become pregnant. Studies have not been done in humans. However, studies in rats receiving doses of 1300 times the recommended human dose and in rabbits receiving 165 times the recommended dose have shown a decrease in successful pregnancies. Terazosin has not been shown to cause birth defects in rats or rabbits.

—if you are **breast-feeding**. It is not known whether terazosin passes into the breast milk. However, this medicine has not been shown to cause problems in nursing babies.

—if you are taking **any** other prescription or nonprescription (OTC) medicine.

Proper Use of This Medicine

Importance of diet—When prescribing medicine for your condition, your doctor may also prescribe a personal diet for you. Such a diet may be low in sodium (salt). Most people eat much more sodium than they need and too much sodium in the diet may increase blood pressure. Some foods that contain large amounts of sodium are canned soup, pickles, ketchup, green and ripe olives, relish, frankfurters, soy sauce, and carbonated beverages. Your doctor may want you to limit the amounts of these and other high-sodium foods in your diet. High blood pressure medicine is usually more effective when such a diet is properly followed.

Also, it may be very important for you to go on a reducing diet. However, check with your doctor before changing your diet.

Many patients who have high blood pressure will not notice any signs of the problem. In fact, many may feel normal. It is very important that you **take your medicine exactly as directed** and that you keep your appointments with your doctor even if you feel well.

Remember that terazosin will not cure your high blood pressure but it does help control it. Therefore, you must continue to take it as directed if you expect to lower your blood pressure and keep it down. **You may have to take high blood pressure medicine for the rest of your life.** If high blood pressure is not treated, it can cause serious problems such as heart failure, blood vessel disease, stroke, or kidney disease.

To help you remember to take your medicine, try to get into the habit of taking it at the same time each day.

If you miss a dose of this medicine, take it as soon as possible the same day. However, if you do not remember the missed dose until the next day, skip the missed dose and go back to your regular dosing schedule. Do not double doses.

How to store this medicine:

- **Keep out of the reach of children.**

- Store away from heat and direct light.

- Do not store in the bathroom, near the kitchen sink, or in other damp places. Heat or moisture may cause the medicine to break down.

- Do not keep outdated medicine or medicine no longer needed. Be sure that any discarded medicine is out of the reach of children.

Precautions While Using This Medicine

It is important that your doctor check your progress at regular visits to make sure that this medicine is working properly.

Do not take other medicines unless they have been discussed with your doctor. This especially includes over-the-counter (nonprescription) medicines for appetite control, asthma, colds, cough, hay fever, or sinus problems, since they may tend to increase your blood pressure.

Dizziness, drowsiness, and irregular heartbeat may occur while you are taking terazosin. These effects are more likely to occur when you first start taking the medicine or when the dosage is increased. To help prevent problems:

—Take the first dose at bedtime. However, **be especially careful if you need to get up during the night.**

—**Make sure you know how you react to this medicine before you drive, use machines, or do other jobs that could be dangerous if you are not alert.**

After you have taken several doses of terazosin, these effects should lessen.

Dizziness, lightheadedness, or fainting may occur while you are being treated with terazosin, especially when you get up from a lying or sitting position. Getting up slowly may help lessen this problem. **If you begin to feel dizzy, lie down so that you do not faint.** Then sit for a few moments before standing to prevent the dizziness from returning.

The dizziness, lightheadedness, or fainting is also more likely to occur if you drink alcohol, stand for long periods of time, exercise, or if the weather is hot. **While you are taking this medicine, be careful in the amount of alcohol you drink. Also, use extra care during exercise or hot weather or if you must stand for long periods of time.**

Side Effects of This Medicine

Along with its needed effects, a medicine may cause some unwanted effects. Although not all of these side effects may occur, if they do occur they may need medical attention.

Check with your doctor as soon as possible if any of the following side effects occur:

More common
> Dizziness or lightheadedness, especially when getting up from a lying or sitting position

Less common
> Chest pain
> Fainting (sudden)
> Fast or irregular heartbeat
> Swelling of feet or lower legs

Rare
> Weight gain

Other side effects may occur that usually do not require medical attention. These side effects may go away during treatment as your body adjusts to the medicine. However, check with your doctor if any of the following side effects continue or are bothersome:

More common
> Headache
> Unusual tiredness or weakness

Less common
> Back or joint pain
> Blurred vision
> Drowsiness
> Nausea and vomiting
> Stuffy nose

For elderly patients:

• Some medicines may affect older patients differently than they do younger adults. Dizziness, lightheadedness, or fainting may be more likely to occur in the elderly, who are more sensitive to the effects of terazosin. In addition, terazosin may reduce tolerance to cold temperatures in elderly patients. Check with your doctor if any of these effects continue or are bothersome. In addition, it is a good idea to check with your doctor or pharmacist if you notice any other unusual effects while taking this medicine or if you think it is not working as it should.

Other side effects not listed above may also occur in some patients. If you notice any other effects, check with your doctor.

Glossary

Abortifacient—Medicine that causes abortion.

Abrade—Scrape or rub away the external surface.

Achlorhydria—Absence of acid in the stomach.

Acidifier, urinary—Medicine that makes the urine more acidic.

Acidosis—Build-up of too much acid in the blood and body fluids and tissues.

Acromegaly—Increase in size of the face, hands, and feet because of too much growth hormone.

Addison's disease—Disease caused by not enough secretion of hormones by the adrenal glands.

Adhesion—The union by connective tissue of two parts that are normally separate (such as parts of a joint).

Adjunct medicine—Medicine always used with another medicine or procedure for treatment of a particular condition; not effective for that condition if used alone. Also called adjuvant medicine.

Adrenal cortex—Outer layer of tissue of the adrenal gland, which produces hormones.

Adrenal glands—Two triangle-shaped organs located next to the kidneys. They produce several important substances necessary for healthy body functioning.

Adrenocorticoid—Hormone produced naturally by the adrenal glands and necessary to maintain good health. Certain adrenocorticoids also are used to provide relief for inflamed areas of the body and as part of the treatment for a number of different diseases, such as severe allergies or skin problems, asthma, or arthritis. Some of the adrenocorticoids used as medicine are the same as those produced naturally by the body.

African sleeping sickness—See Trypanosomiasis, African.

Agoraphobia—Fear of public places or open spaces.

AIDS (acquired immune deficiency syndrome)—Disease caused by the HIV virus which results in a breakdown of the body's immune system, thereby making a person more susceptible to other infections and some forms of cancer.

Alcohol-abuse deterrent—Medicine used to help alcoholics avoid the use of alcohol.

Alkalizer, urinary—Medicine used to make the urine more alkaline.

Altitude sickness agent—Medicine used to prevent or lessen some of the effects of high altitude on the body.

Alzheimer's disease—Progressive disorder of thinking and other mental processes, usually associated with age.

Aminoglycoside—A class of chemically related antibiotics used to treat some serious types of bacterial infections.

Anabolic steroids—Substances produced by the body that promote the growth of body tissue.

Analgesic—Medicine that relieves pain without causing unconsciousness.

Anaphylaxis—Sudden, severe allergic reaction.

Androgen—Male hormone.

Anemia—Too little hemoglobin in the blood, resulting in tiredness, breathlessness, and poor resistance to infection.

Anesthesiologist—A physician who is qualified to give an anesthetic and other medicines to a patient before and during surgery.

Anesthetic—Medicine that causes a loss of sensation of pain, sometimes through loss of consciousness.

Angina—Pain, tightness, or feeling of heaviness in the chest, sometimes accompanied by difficulty in breathing. The pain may be felt in the left shoulder and arm instead of or in addition to the chest. These symptoms often occur during exercise.

Angioedema—Allergic condition marked by continuing swelling and severe itching of areas of the skin.

Antacid—Medicine used to neutralize excess acid in the stomach.

Anthelmintic—Medicine used to treat infections caused by worms.

Antiacne agent—Medicine used to treat acne.

Antiadrenal—Medicine used to prevent an overactive adrenal gland (adrenal cortex) from producing too much cortisone-like hormone.

Antianemic—Medicine to treat anemia.

Antianginal—Medicine used to prevent or treat angina attacks.

Antianxiety agent—Medicine used for the treatment of nervousness, tension, or excessive anxiety.

Antiarrhythmic—Medicine used to treat irregular heartbeats.

Antiasthmatic—Medicine used to treat asthma.

Antibacterial—Medicine that destroys bacteria or suppresses their growth.

Antibiotic—Medicine produced by micro-organisms and used to treat various types of infections.

Antibody—Special kind of blood protein that helps the body fight infection.

Anticholelithic—Medicine that dissolves gallstones.

Anticoagulant—Medicine that prevents blood clots from being formed in the blood vessels.

Anticonvulsant—Medicine used to prevent or treat convulsions (seizures).

Antidepressant—Medicine used to treat mental depression.

Antidiabetic agent—Medicine used to control blood sugar levels in patients with diabetes mellitus (sugar diabetes).

Antidiarrheal—Medicine used to treat diarrhea.

Antidiuretic—Medicine used to help hold water in the body (for example, in patients with diabetes insipidus [water diabetes]).

Antidote—Medicine used for preventing or treating harmful effects of another medicine or a poison.

Antidyskinetic—Medicine used in the treatment of certain diseases that cause a loss of muscle control.

Antidysmenorrheal—Medicine used to treat menstrual cramps.

Antiemetic—Medicine used to prevent or treat nausea and vomiting.

Antienuretic—Medicine used to help prevent bedwetting.

Antifibrotic—Medicine used to treat fibrosis.

Antiflatulent—Medicine used to help relieve excess gas in the stomach or intestines.

Antifungal—Medicine used to treat infections caused by a fungus.

Antiglaucoma agent—Medicine used to treat glaucoma.

Antigout agent—Medicine used to prevent or relieve gout attacks.

Antihemorrhagic—Medicine used to prevent or help stop serious bleeding.

Antihistaminic, H_1-receptor—Medicine used to prevent or relieve the symptoms of allergies (such as hay fever).

Antihypercalcemic—Medicine used to help lower the amount of calcium in the blood.

Antihyperlipidemic—Medicine used to help lower the amount of cholesterol or other fat-like substances in the blood.

Antihypertensive—Medicine used in the treatment of high blood pressure.

Antihyperuricemic—Medicine used to prevent or treat gout or other medical problems caused by too much uric acid in the blood.

Antihypocalcemic—Medicine used to increase calcium levels in patients with too little calcium.

Antihypoglycemic—Medicine used to increase blood sugar levels in patients with low blood sugar.

Antihypokalemic—Medicine used to increase potassium levels in patients with too little potassium.

Antihypoparathyroid—Medicine used to treat the effects of an underactive parathyroid gland.

Anti-infective—Medicine that fights infection.

Anti-inflammatory—Medicine used to relieve pain, swelling, and other symptoms caused by inflammation.

Anti-inflammatory, nonsteroidal—An anti-inflammatory medicine that is not a cortisone-like medicine.

Anti-inflammatory, steroidal—A cortisone-like anti-inflammatory medicine.

Antimanic—Medicine used to treat manic-depressive mental illness.

Antimetabolite—Medicine that interferes with the normal processes within cells, preventing their growth.

Antimuscarinic—Medicine used to block the effects of a certain chemical in the body; often used to reduce smooth muscle spasms, especially abdominal or stomach cramps or spasms. It is also used to help reduce the amount of stomach acid.

Antimyasthenic—Medicine used in the treatment of myasthenia gravis.

Antimyotonic—Medicine used to prevent or relieve nighttime leg cramps or muscle spasms.

Antineoplastic—Medicine that is used to treat cancer.

Antineuralgic—Medicine used to treat neuralgia.

Antiprotozoal—Medicine used to treat infections caused by protozoa (tiny, one-celled animals).

Antipsoriatic—Medicine used to treat psoriasis.

Antipsychotic—Medicine used to treat certain nervous, mental, and emotional conditions.

Antipyretic—Medicine used to reduce high fever.

Antirheumatic—Medicine used to treat arthritis (rheumatism).

Antiseborrheic—Medicine used to treat dandruff and seborrhea.

Antiseptic—Medicine that fights bacteria and is used to clean objects or surfaces and thereby prevent infections.

Antispasmodic—Medicine used to reduce smooth muscle spasms (for example, stomach, intestinal, or urinary tract spasms).

Antispastic—Medicine used to treat muscle spasms.

Antithyroid agent—Medicine used to treat the effects of an overactive thyroid gland.

Antitremor agent—Medicine used to treat tremors (trembling or shaking).

Antitubercular—Medicine used to treat tuberculosis (TB).

Antitussive—Medicine used to relieve cough.

Antiulcer agent—Medicine used in the treatment of stomach and duodenal ulcers.

Antivertigo agent—Medicine used to prevent dizziness.

Antiviral—Medicine used to treat infections caused by a virus.

Apoplexy—See Stroke.

Appendicitis—Inflammation of the appendix.

Appetite stimulant—Medicine used to help increase the appetite.

Appetite suppressant—Medicine used in weight control programs to help decrease the desire for food.

ARC (AIDS-related complex)—Thought to be a forerunner of AIDS. Refers to certain conditions caused by the AIDS virus. Although not AIDS itself, the symptoms of ARC are usually the same as those of AIDS.

Arteritis, temporal—Inflammatory disease of the blood vessels, usually of the scalp, occurring in the elderly.

Arthritis, rheumatoid—Chronic disease of the joints, marked by pain and swelling at the sites.

Asthma—Lung condition marked by spasms of the bronchial tubes (air passages), which prevent normal breathing and air exchange.

Bacterium—Tiny, one-celled organism. Many types of bacteria are responsible for a number of diseases and infections.

Beriberi—Disorder caused by too little vitamin B_1 (thiamine), marked by an accumulation of fluid in the body, extreme weight loss, inflammation of nerves, or paralysis.

Bile—Thick fluid produced by the liver and stored in the gallbladder. Bile helps in the digestion of food.

Bile duct—Tubular passage through which bile passes from the liver to the gallbladder.

Bilharziasis—See Manson's schistosomiasis.

Biliary—Relating to bile, the bile duct, or the gallbladder.

Bipolar disorder—Also called manic-depressive illness. Severe mental illness marked by repeated episodes of depression, mania, or both.

Black fever—See Leishmaniasis, visceral.

Blood fluke—See Manson's schistosomiasis.

Bone resorption inhibitor—Medicine used to prevent or treat certain types of bone disorders, such as Paget's disease of the bone.

Bowel disease, inflammatory, suppressant—Medicine used to treat certain types of intestinal disorders, such as colitis.

Bradycardia—Slowing of the heart rate to fewer than 50 beats per minute.

Bronchitis—Inflammation of the bronchial tubes (air passages).

Bronchodilator—Medicine used to open up the bronchial tubes (air passages) of the lungs to increase the flow of air through them.

Buccal—Relating to the cheek. A buccal medicine is taken by placing it in the cheek pocket and letting it slowly dissolve.

Bursa—Small sac of tissue present where body parts move over one another (such as a joint) to help reduce friction.

Bursitis—Inflammation of a bursa.

Candidiasis of the mouth—See Thrush.

Cardiac—Relating to the heart.

Cardiac load–reducing agent—Medicine used to ease the workload of the heart by allowing the blood to flow through the body more easily.

Cardiotonic—Medicine used to improve the strength and efficiency of the heart.

Caries, dental—Also called "cavities." Tooth decay causing pain and leading to the crumbling of the tooth.

Cataract—An opacity (cloudiness) in the eye or lens that impairs vision or causes blindness.

Catheter—Tube to be inserted into a small opening in the body so that fluids can be put in or taken out.

Caustic—Burning or corrosive agent. Medicine applied to the skin to remove calluses, corns, and warts.

Cavities—See Caries, dental.

Cerebral palsy—Brain condition resulting in weakness and poor coordination of the limbs.

Chickenpox—See Varicella.

Cholelitholytic—Medicine used to dissolve gallstones.

Cholesterol—Fat-like material found in the blood and most tissues. Too much cholesterol is associated with several potential health risks, especially atherosclerosis (hardening of the arteries).

Chronic—Describing a condition of long duration, involving very slow changes, and often of gradual onset. Note that the term "chronic" has nothing to do with how serious the condition is.

Cirrhosis—Liver disease marked by abnormal cell growth, which may in turn lead to other serious conditions.

Cold sores—See Herpes simplex.

Colitis—Inflammation of the colon (bowel).

Colostomy—Operation in which part of the colon (bowel) is brought through the abdominal wall and opened so as to drain the intestine, thus bypassing the rest of the intestines.

Coma—State of unconsciousness from which the patient cannot be aroused.

Coma, hepatic—Disturbances in mental function and the nervous system caused by severe liver disease.

Conjunctiva—Delicate mucous membrane covering the front of the eye and the inside of the eyelid.

Conjunctivitis—Inflammation of the conjunctiva.

Contraceptive—Medicine or device used to prevent pregnancy.

Cot death—See Sudden infant death syndrome (SIDS).

Cowpox—See Vaccinia.

Creutzfeldt-Jakob disease—Rare disease, probably caused by a slow-acting virus that affects the brain and nervous system.

Crib death—See Sudden infant death syndrome (SIDS).

Crohn's disease—Condition in which parts of the digestive tract become thick and inflamed.

Croup—Inflammation and blockage of the larynx (voice box) in young children.

Cushing's syndrome—Condition in which the adrenal gland produces too much cortisone-like hormone, leading to weight gain, round face, and high blood pressure.

Cycloplegia—Paralysis of certain eye muscles, which can be useful in resting the muscles.

Cycloplegic—Medicine used to induce cycloplegia.

Cyst—Abnormal sac or closed cavity filled with liquid or semisolid matter.

Cystic—Marked by cysts.

Cystitis, interstitial—Inflammation of the bladder, predominantly in women, with frequent urge to urinate and painful urination.

Decongestant, nasal—Medicine used to help relieve nasal congestion (stuffy nose).

Decongestant, ophthalmic—Medicine used in the eye to relieve redness, burning, itching, or other irritation.

Dental—Related to the teeth or gums.

Depression, mental—Deep sadness and difficulty in performing day-to-day tasks. Other symptoms include disturbances in sleep, appetite, and concentration.

Dermatitis herpetiformis—Skin disease marked by sores and itching.

Dermatitis, seborrheic—Type of eczema found on the scalp and face.

Dermatomyositis—Inflammatory disorder of the skin and underlying tissues, including breakdown of muscle fibers.

Diabetes insipidus—Also called "water diabetes." Disorder in which the patient produces large amounts of urine and is constantly thirsty.

Diabetes mellitus—Also called "sugar diabetes." Disorder in which the body cannot process sugars to produce energy, due to lack of the hormone called insulin. This leads to too much sugar in the blood (hyperglycemia).

Dialysis, renal—Artificial technique for removing waste materials or poisons from the blood when the kidneys are not working properly.

Digestant—Medicine used to help the stomach digest food.

Diuretic—Also called "water pill." Medicine that increases the amount of urine produced by helping the kidneys get rid of water and salt.

Diverticulitis—Inflammation of a diverticulum (sac or pouch formed at weak points in the digestive tract).

Down's syndrome—Also called "mongolism." Mental retardation caused by a defect in the genes. Patients with Down's syndrome are marked physically by a round head, flat nose, slightly slanted eyes, and short stature.

Dumdum fever—See Leishmaniasis, visceral.

Duodenum—First of the three parts of the small intestine.

Eczema—Inflammation of the skin, marked by itching and rash.

Edema—Swelling of body tissue due to accumulation of fluids, usually first observed in the feet or lower legs.

Eighth-cranial-nerve disease—Disease of the eighth cranial (brain) nerve, resulting in dizziness, loss of balance, loss of hearing, nausea, or vomiting.

Emollient—Substance that soothes and softens an irritated surface, such as the skin.

Emphysema—Lung condition in which too much air accumulates in lung tissue because of blockage or narrowing of the bronchial tubes (air passages), leading to troubled breathing and heart problems.

Encephalitis—Inflammation of the brain.

Encephalopathy—Any of a group of diseases that affect the brain.

Endocarditis—Inflammation of the lining of the heart, leading to fever, heart murmurs, and heart failure.

Endometriosis—Condition in which material similar to the lining of the womb appears at other sites within the pelvic cavity, causing pain and bleeding.

Enteric coating—Coating on tablets which allows them to pass through the stomach unchanged before being broken up in the intestine and being absorbed. Used to protect the stomach from the drug and/or the drug from the stomach's acid.

Enteritis—Inflammation of the small intestine, usually causing diarrhea.

Enuresis—Urinating while asleep (bedwetting).

Enzyme—Type of protein produced by living cells that is important for normal chemical reactions in the body.

Epidural space—Area in the spinal column into which medicines (usually for pain) can be administered.

Epilepsy—Any of a group of brain disorders featuring sudden attacks of seizures and other symptoms.

Ergot alkaloids—Medicines that cause narrowing of blood vessels; used to treat migraine headaches, and to reduce bleeding in childbirth.

Estrogen—Female hormone necessary for the normal sexual development of the female and for the regulation of the menstrual cycle during the childbearing years.

Expectorant—Medicine used to relieve cough by loosening and thinning the mucus or phlegm in the lungs so that it may be coughed up.

Familial Mediterranean fever—Also called polyserositis. Inherited condition involving inflammation of the lining of the chest, abdomen, and joints.

Favism—Inherited allergy to broad (fava) beans.

Fibrocystic—Having benign (noncancerous) tumors of connective tissue.

Fibrosis—Condition in which the skin and underlying tissues tighten and become less flexible.

Fibrosis, cystic—Disease in which abnormally thick mucus is produced, which interferes with a number of important organs, and often leads to infections of the lungs.

Flu—See Influenza.

Gamma globulin—Type of protein found in the blood that is important in the body's immunity to infection.

Gastric—Relating to the stomach.

Gastric acid secretion inhibitor—Medicine used to decrease the amount of acid formed by the stomach.

Gastroenteritis—Inflammation of the stomach and intestine.

Gastroparesis, diabetic—Condition brought on by diabetes in which the stomach does not function as it should.

Generic—General in nature; relating to an entire group or class. In relation to medicines, the general name of a drug substance; not owned by one specific group as would be true for a trademark or brand name.

Gilles de la Tourette syndrome—See Tourette's disorder.

Gingiva—Gums.

Gingival hyperplasia—Enlargement of the gums.

Gingivitis—Inflammation of the gums.

Glandular fever—See Mononucleosis.

Glaucoma—Condition in which loss of vision may occur because of abnormally high pressure in the eye.

Glucose-6-phosphate dehydrogenase (G6PD) deficiency—Lack of or reduced amounts of an enzyme (glucose-6-phosphate dehydrogenase) that breaks down certain sugar compounds in the body.

Gluten—Type of protein found especially in wheat and rye.

Goiter—Enlargement of the thyroid gland that causes the neck to swell. Condition results from a lack of iodine or thyroid hormone.

Gonadotropin—Hormone that stimulates the actions of the sex organs.

Gout—Disease in which too much uric acid builds up in the blood and joints, leading to painful swelling.

Graves' disease—Disorder in which too much thyroid hormone is present in the blood.

Guillain-Barré syndrome—Nerve disease marked by sudden numbness and weakness in the limbs that may progress to complete paralysis.

Hair follicle—Sheath of tissue surrounding a hair root.

Hansen's disease—See Leprosy.

Hartnup disease—Hereditary disease in which the body has trouble processing certain chemicals, leading to mental retardation, rough skin, and problems with muscle coordination.

Heart attack—See Myocardial infarction.

Hemoglobin—Iron-containing substance found in red blood cells that transports oxygen from the lungs to the tissues of the body.

Hemolytic anemia—Type of anemia caused by destruction of red blood cells.

Hemophilia—Hereditary blood disease in males in which blood clotting is delayed, leading to excessive and uncontrolled bleeding even after minor injuries.

Hemorrhoids—Also called "piles." Enlarged veins in the walls of the anus.

Hepatic—Relating to the liver.

Hepatitis—Inflammation of the liver.

Hernia, hiatal—Condition in which the stomach passes partly into the chest through the opening for the esophagus in the diaphragm.

Herpes simplex—Also called "cold sores." Inflammation of the skin, caused by a virus, resulting in groups of small, painful blisters. They may occur either around the mouth or, in the case of genital herpes, around the genitals (sex organs).

Herpes zoster—Also called "shingles." Inflammation of the nerves, caused by a virus, usually marked by pain and blisters on the face, chest, or stomach. The virus that causes herpes zoster also causes chickenpox.

High blood pressure—See Hypertension.

Hodgkin's disease—Malignant condition marked by swelling of the lymph glands, with weight loss and fever.

Hormone—Substance produced in one part of the body (such as a gland) which then passes into the bloodstream and is carried to other organs or tissues, where it helps them to function.

Hyperactivity—Abnormally increased activity.

Hypercalcemia—Too much calcium in the blood.

Hypercalciuria—Too much calcium in the urine.

Hyperglycemia—High blood sugar.

Hyperphosphatemia—Too much phosphate in the blood.

Hypertension—Also called "high blood pressure." Blood pressure in the arteries (blood vessels) that is higher than normal for the patient's age group. Hypertension often shows no outward signs or symptoms but may lead to a number of serious health problems.

Hyperthermia—Very high body temperature.

Hypocalcemia—Too little calcium in the blood.

Hypoglycemia—Low blood sugar.

Hypothalamus—Area of the brain that controls a number of body functions, including temperature, thirst, hunger, sexual and emotional activity, and sleep.

Ileostomy—Operation in which the ileum is brought through the abdominal wall to create an artificial opening through which the contents of the intestine can be discharged, thus bypassing the colon (bowel).

Ileum—Lowest of the three portions of the small intestine.

Immune system—Defense network of the body, designed to destroy anything "foreign" in the body.

Immunizing agent, active—Agent that causes the body to produce its own antibodies for protection against certain infections.

Immunosuppressant—Medicine that reduces the body's natural immunity.

Infertility—Inability of a woman to become pregnant or of a man to cause pregnancy.

Inflammation—Pain, redness, swelling, and heat in a part of the body, usually in response to injury or illness.

Influenza—Also called "flu." Highly contagious virus infection of the lungs, marked by coughing and sneezing, headache, chills, fever, muscle pain, and general weakness.

Inhalation—Medicine used by being breathed in (inhaled) into the lungs. Some inhalations work locally in the lungs, while others produce their effects elsewhere in the body.

Inhibitor—Substance that prevents a process or reaction.

Interstitial plasma cell pneumonia—See Pneumocystis pneumonia.

Intra-amniotic—Within the sac that contains the fetus and amniotic fluid.

Intra-arterial—Into an artery.

Intracavernosal—Into the corpus cavernosa (cavities in the penis that, when filled with blood, produce an erection).

Intracavitary—Into a body cavity (for example, the chest cavity or bladder).

Intramuscular—Into a muscle.

Intrauterine device (IUD)—Small plastic or metal device placed in the uterus (womb) to prevent pregnancy.

Intravenous—Into a vein.

Irrigation—Washing out a body cavity or wound with a solution of a medicine.

Jaundice—Yellowing of the eyes and skin due to too much of a certain pigment in the bile.

Kala-azar—See Leishmaniasis, visceral.

Keratolytic—Medicine used to soften hardened areas of the skin (e.g., warts).

Ketoacidosis—Type of acidosis associated with diabetes.

Lactation—Secretion of milk by the mammary glands (breasts).

Larvae—Young or immature insects.

Laxative—Medicine taken to encourage bowel movements.

Laxative, bulk-forming—Laxative that acts by absorbing liquid in the intestines and swelling to form a soft, bulky stool. The bowel is then stimulated normally by the presence of the bulky mass.

Laxative, hyperosmotic—Laxative that acts by drawing water into the bowel from surrounding body tissues. This provides a soft stool mass and increased bowel action.

Laxative, lubricant—Laxative that acts by coating the bowel and the stool mass with a waterproof film. This keeps moisture in the stool. The stool remains soft and its passage is made easier.

Laxative, stimulant—Also called contact laxative. Laxative that acts directly on the intestinal wall. The direct stimulation increases the muscle contractions that move along the stool mass.

Laxative, stool softener—Also called emollient laxative. Laxative that acts by helping liquids mix into the stool and prevent dry, hard stool masses. The stool remains soft and its passage is made easier.

Legionnaires' disease—Lung infection caused by a certain bacterium.

Leishmaniasis, visceral—Also called "black fever," "Dumdum fever," or "kala-azar." Tropical disease, transmitted by sandfly bites, which causes liver and spleen enlargement, anemia, weight loss, and fever.

Leprosy—Also called "Hansen's disease." Chronic disease affecting the skin, mucous membranes, and nerves. Symptoms include severe numbness, weakness, and paralysis leading to disfigurement and deformity.

Leukemia—Disease of the blood and bone marrow in which too many white blood cells are produced, resulting in anemia, bleeding, and low resistance to infections.

Leukoderma—See Vitiligo.

Lugol's solution—Transparent, deep brown liquid containing iodine and potassium iodide, which may be given before a radiopharmaceutical medicine.

Lupus—See Lupus erythematosus.

Lupus erythematosus, systemic—Also called "lupus" or "SLE (Systemic Lupus Erythematosus)." Chronic inflammatory disease affecting the skin and various internal organs.

Lymph—Fluid that bathes the tissues. It is derived from blood and circulated by the lymphatic system.

Lymphatic system—Network of vessels that conveys lymph from the tissue fluids to the bloodstream.

Lymph node—Filter through which lymph passes as it circulates throughout the lymphatic system.

Macrobiotic—Vegetarian diet consisting mostly of whole grains.

Malignant—Describing a condition that becomes continually worse if untreated; also used to mean cancerous.

Malnutrition—Condition caused by unbalanced or insufficient diet.

Mammogram—X-ray picture of the breast, usually taken to check for abnormal growths.

Mania—Mental state of unusual cheerfulness and activity, but marked by illogical thought and speech, and overbearing, often violent behavior.

Manson's schistosomiasis—Also called "blood fluke" or "bilharziasis." Tropical infection in which worms enter the body from contaminated water and settle in the intestines, causing anemia and inflammation.

Mast cell—Large cell that releases certain substances that cause allergic reactions.

Mastocytosis—Accumulation of too many mast cells in the tissues in infants, resulting in a distinctive skin rash.

Megavitamin therapy—Taking very large doses of vitamins to prevent or treat certain medical problems. Studies have not proven this to be useful.

Melanoma—Highly malignant cancer tumor, usually occurring on the skin.

Meningitis—Inflammation of the tissues that surround the brain and spinal cord.

Migraine—Throbbing headache caused by enlarged blood vessels, usually affecting one side of the head.

Miotic—Medicine used in the eye that causes the pupil to constrict (become smaller).

Mongolism—See Down's syndrome.

Mono—See Mononucleosis.

Monoclonal—Derived from a single cell; related to production of drugs by genetic engineering (e.g., monoclonal antibodies).

Mononucleosis—Also called "mono" or "glandular fever." Infectious viral disease occurring mostly in adolescents and young adults, marked by swelling of the lymph nodes in the neck, armpits, and groin, and by severe fatigue.

Mucolytic—Medicine that breaks down or dissolves mucus.

Mucosal—Relating to the mucous membrane.

Mucous membrane—Moist layer of tissue surrounding or lining many body structures and cavities, including the mouth, lips, and inside of nose.

Mucus—Thick fluid produced by the body as a protective barrier, as a lubricant, and as a carrier of enzymes.

Multiple sclerosis (MS)—Chronic, progressive nerve disease marked by unsteadiness, shakiness, and problems in speech.

Myasthenia gravis—Chronic disease marked by abnormal weakness, and sometimes paralysis, of certain muscles.

Mydriatic—Medicine used in the eye that causes the pupil to dilate (become larger).

Myelogram—X-ray picture of the spinal cord.

Myeloma, multiple—Cancerous bone marrow disease that affects the body's ability to fight infections.

Myocardial infarction—Also called "heart attack." Interruption of blood supply to the heart, leading to sudden, severe chest pain, and damage to the heart muscle.

Myocardial reinfarction prophylactic—Medicine used to help prevent additional heart attacks in patients who have already had one attack.

Myotonia congenita—Hereditary muscle disorder marked by difficulty in relaxing a muscle or releasing a grip after any strong effort.

Narcolepsy—Extreme tendency to fall asleep suddenly.

Nasal—Relating to the nose.

Nasogastric (NG) tube—Tube that is inserted through the nose, down the throat, and into the stomach, so that medicine, food, or nutrients may be administered to patients who cannot swallow.

Nebulizer—Instrument that applies liquid in the form of a fine spray.

Neuralgia—Pain along the course of one or more nerves, occurring suddenly and intensely.

Neuralgia, trigeminal—Also called "tic douloureux." Severe burning or stabbing pain along the nerves in the face.

Neuritis, optic—Disease of the nerves in the eye.

Nicotinamide adenine dinucleotide (NADH) methemoglobin reductase deficiency—Reduced ability of the blood to carry oxygen caused by the lack of or reduced amount of a specific enzyme.

Nonsuppurative—Not discharging pus.

Obesity—Accumulation of excess fat.

Obstetrics—Area of medicine concerned with the care of women during pregnancy and childbirth.

Occlusive dressing—Dressing (such as plastic kitchen wrap) that completely cuts off air to the skin.

Ophthalmic—Relating to the eye.

Orchitis—Inflammation of the testis.

Osteitis deformans—See Paget's disease.

Osteomalacia—Softening of the bones due to lack of vitamin D.

Osteoporosis—Loss of bone tissue, resulting in bones that are brittle and easily fractured.

Otic—Relating to the ear.

Paget's disease—Also called "osteitis deformans." Chronic bone disease, marked by thickening of the bones and severe pain.

Pancreatitis—Inflammation of the pancreas.

Paralysis agitans—See Parkinson's disease.

Parkinsonism—See Parkinson's disease.

Parkinson's disease—Also called "Parkinsonism," "paralysis agitans," or "shaking palsy." Brain disease marked by tremor (shaking), stiffness, and difficulty in moving.

Patent ductus arteriosus (PDA)—Condition in newborn babies in which an important blood vessel in the heart fails to close as it should, resulting in faulty circulation and serious health problems.

Pediculicide—Medicine that kills lice.

Pellagra—Disease caused by too little vitamin B_3 (niacin), resulting in scaly skin, diarrhea, and mental depression.

Pemphigus—Skin disease marked by successive outbreaks of blisters.

Peritoneum—Sac that contains the liver, stomach, and intestines.

Peyronie's disease—Dense, fiber-like growth in the penis, which can be felt as an irregular hard lump, and which usually causes bending and pain when the penis is erect.

Phenol—Substance used as a preservative for injections.

Pheochromocytoma (PCC)—Small tumor of the adrenal gland.

Phlebitis—Inflammation of a vein.

Piles—See Hemorrhoids.

Pituitary gland—Pea-sized body located at the base of the skull. It produces a number of hormones that are essential to normal body growth and functioning.

Placebo—Also called "sugar pill." Medicine that has no actual effect on the patient but may help to relieve a condition because the patient believes it will.

Plaque—Mixture of saliva, bacteria, and carbohydrates that forms on the teeth, leading to caries (cavities) and other dental problems.

Platelet—Disc-shaped structure in the blood which performs several functions relating to blood clotting.

Platelet aggregation inhibitor—Medicine used to help prevent the platelets in the blood from clumping together. This effect reduces the chance of heart attack or stroke in certain patients.

Pleura—Membrane covering the lungs.

Pneumococcal—Relating to certain bacteria that cause pneumonia.

Pneumocystis pneumonia—Also called "interstitial plasma cell pneumonia." A very serious type of pneumonia usually affecting infants and patients in a weakened condition.

Polymorphous light eruption—A skin problem in certain people resulting from exposure to sunlight.

Polymyalgia rheumatica—Rheumatic disease, most common in elderly patients, that causes aching and stiffness in the shoulders and hips.

Polyp—Swollen or tumorous tissue which may or may not be cancerous.

Porphyria—Rare, inherited blood disease.

Priapism—Prolonged abnormal, painful erection of the penis.

Proctitis—Inflammation of the rectum.

Progestin—Female hormone necessary during the childbearing years for the development of the milk-producing glands, and for the proper regulation of the menstrual cycle.

Prolactinoma—Pituitary tumor.

Prophylactic—1. Used to prevent the occurrence of a specific condition. 2. Condom.

Prosthesis—Any artificial substitute for a missing body part.

Protozoa—Tiny, one-celled animals, some of which are important disease-causing parasites in man.

Psoralen—Chemical found in plants and used in certain perfumes and medicines. Exposure to a psoralen and then to sunlight may increase the risk of severe burning.

Psoriasis—Chronic skin disease marked by itchy, scaly, red patches.

Psychosis—Severe mental illness marked by loss of contact with reality, often involving delusions, hallucinations, and disordered thinking.

PUVA—The combination of a psoralen, such as methoxsalen or trioxsalen, and ultraviolet light A; used to treat psoriasis and some other skin conditions.

Rachischisis—See Spina bifida.

Radiopaque agent—Substance that makes it easier to see an area of the body with x-rays. Radiopaque agents are used to help diagnose a variety of medical problems.

Radiopharmaceutical—Radioactive agent used to diagnose certain medical problems or treat certain diseases.

Raynaud's syndrome—Condition marked by paleness, numbness, and discomfort in the fingers when they are exposed to cold.

Rectal—Relating to the rectum.

Renal—Relating to the kidneys.

Reye's syndrome—Serious disease affecting the liver and brain that sometimes occurs after a virus infection such as flu or chickenpox. It occurs most often in young children and teenagers. The first sign of Reye's syndrome is usually severe, prolonged vomiting.

Rheumatic heart disease—Heart disease marked by scarring and chronic inflammation of the heart and its valves, occurring after rheumatic fever.

Rhinitis—Inflammation of the mucous membrane inside the nose.

Rickets—Bone disease resulting in soft and malformed bones; caused by too little vitamin D.

Ringworm—See Tinea.

Sarcoidosis—Chronic disorder in which the lymph nodes in many parts of the body are enlarged, and small fleshy swellings develop in the lungs, liver, and spleen.

Scabicide—Medicine used to treat scabies (itch mite) infection.

Scabies—Skin infection caused by a mite, resulting in severe itching and redness.

Schizophrenia—Severe mental disorder marked by a breakdown of the thinking process, of contact with reality, and of normal emotional responses.

Scintigram—Image obtained by detecting radiation emitted from a radiopharmaceutical introduced into the body.

Scleroderma—Persistent hardening and shrinking of the body's connective tissue.

Scrotum—Sac that holds the testes (male sex glands).

Scurvy—Disease caused by too little vitamin C (ascorbic acid), marked by bleeding gums, bleeding beneath the skin, and impaired healing of wounds.

Secretion—1. Process in which a gland releases a substance into the body for use. 2. The substance released by the gland.

Sedative-hypnotic—Medicine used to treat nervousness, restlessness, or insomnia (sleeplessness).

Shaking palsy—See Parkinson's disease.

Shingles—See Herpes simplex.

Shunt—Surgical tube used to transfer blood from one part of the body to another.

SIADH (secretion of inappropriate antidiuretic hormone) syndrome—Disease in which the body retains (keeps) more fluid and loses more sodium than usual.

Sickle cell anemia—Hereditary blood disease that predominantly affects blacks; name comes from the sickle-shaped red blood cells found in the blood of patients.

Sinusitis—Inflammation of a sinus.

Sjögren's syndrome—Condition marked by swollen salivary glands and dryness of the mouth.

Skeletal muscle relaxant—Medicine used to relax certain muscles and help relieve the pain and discomfort caused by strains, sprains, or other injury to the muscles.

SLE—See Lupus erythematosus.

Spastic paralysis—Weakness of a limb because of too much reflex response.

Spina bifida—Also called "rachischisis." Birth defect in which the infant's spinal cord is partially exposed through a hole in the backbone.

Stimulant, respiratory—Medicine used to stimulate breathing.

Stroke—Also called "apoplexy." Sudden weakness or paralysis, usually affecting one side of the body. Stroke occurs when the flow of blood to an area of the brain is interrupted.

Subcutaneous—Under the skin.

Sublingual—Under the tongue. A sublingual medicine is taken by placing it under the tongue and letting it slowly dissolve.

Sudden infant death syndrome (SIDS)—Also called "crib death" or "cot death." Death of a baby, usually while asleep, from an unknown cause.

Sugar diabetes—See Diabetes mellitus.

Sugar pill—See Placebo.

Sulfite—Type of preservative; causes allergic reactions, such as asthma, in some sensitive patients.

Sulfone—Medicine which acts against the bacteria that cause leprosy and tuberculosis.

Suppository—Cone or cylinder of medicated material for insertion into the rectum or vagina. Suppository is solid at room temperature but melts at body temperature.

Systemic—For general effects throughout the body; applies to most medicines when taken by mouth or given by injection.

Temporomandibular joint (TMJ)—Hinge that connects the lower jaw to the skull.

Tendinitis—Inflammation of a tendon.

Testosterone—Principal male sex hormone.

Therapeutic—Relating to the treatment of a specific condition.

Thimerosal—Chemical used as a preservative in some medicines, and as an antiseptic and disinfectant.

Thrombocytopenic purpura—Blood disease marked by skin rash.

Thrush—Also called "white mouth" or "candidiasis of the mouth." Mild fungal infection of the mouth marked by white patches on the tongue or insides of cheeks.

Thyroid gland—Large gland in the base of the neck. It releases thyroid hormone, which is important for normal body functioning.

Tic—Repeated involuntary movement or spasm of a muscle.

Tic douloureux—See Neuralgia, trigeminal.

Tinea—Also called "ringworm." Fungus infection of the surface of the skin, particularly the scalp, feet, and nails.

Topical—For local effects when applied directly to the skin.

Tourette's disorder—Also called "Gilles de la Tourette syndrome." Condition of severe tics, including vocal tics and involuntary obscene speech.

Toxemia—Blood poisoning caused by bacteria growth at the site of infection.

Toxemia of pregnancy—Disease (of unknown cause) affecting pregnant women.

Toxic—Poisonous; potentially deadly.

Toxoplasmosis—Disease caused by a protozoan; generally the symptoms are mild but a severe lymph node infection can result.

Tracheostomy—A surgical opening through the throat into the trachea (main passage from the lungs to the mouth) to permit a patient to breathe easily.

Transdermal disk—Patch applied to the skin as a means of administering medicine; medicine contained in the patch is absorbed into the body through the skin.

Triglyceride—Substance formed in the body from fat in foods, and used to store fats in blood and tissues.

Trypanosome fever—See Trypanosomiasis, African

Trypanosomiasis, African—Also called "trypanosome fever" or "African sleeping sickness." Tropical disease, transmitted by tsetse fly bites, which causes fever, headache, and chills, followed by enlarged lymph nodes, anemia, and painful limbs and joints. Months or even years later, the disease affects the central nervous system, causing drowsiness and lethargy.

Tuberculosis (TB)—Infectious disease, usually of the lungs, marked by fever, night sweats, weight loss, and spitting up blood.

Ureters—Pair of tubes through which urine passes from the kidneys to the bladder.

Vaccine—Medicine given by mouth or by injection to produce immunity to a certain infection.

Vaccinia—Also called "cowpox." Mild virus infection causing symptoms similar to smallpox.

Vaginal—Relating to the vagina.

Varicella—Also called "chickenpox." Very infectious virus disease marked by fever and itchy rash that develops into blisters and then scabs.

Vascular—Relating to the blood vessels.

Vasodilator—Medicine that dilates the blood vessels, which permits increased blood flow.

Veterinary—Concerning medical care of animals.

Vitiligo—Also called "leukoderma." Condition in which some areas of skin lose their color and turn white.

von Willebrand's disease—Hereditary blood disease in which blood clotting is delayed, leading to excessive and uncontrolled bleeding even after minor injuries.

Water diabetes—See Diabetes insipidus.

Water pill—See Diuretic.

White mouth—See Thrush.

Wilson's disease—Inborn defect in the body's ability to process copper. Too much copper may lead to jaundice, cirrhosis, mental retardation, or symptoms like those of Parkinson's disease.

Zollinger-Ellison syndrome—Disorder in which the stomach produces too much acid, leading to ulcers.

Appendixes

Appendix I: Patient Medication Calendar and Wallet Diary

Filling Out Your Medication Calendar

When filling out the chart for the first time, or when your medication has been changed, you will need the help of your doctor, nurse, or pharmacist. Each month after that, you simply copy the name of the medicine and the strength from the first calendar, following these steps (refer to the numbered arrows in the example):

1. Write in the month that the chart is for.
2. Fill in the days of the week under the right date for that month.
3. Write in the name of your medicine and its strength.
4. Fill in the amount you take at the assigned time.
5. Indicate the hour the medicine should be taken.
6. Place a check in the correct box after you have taken the medicine.

Put the chart where you will see it, such as on the wall or mirror, so it can be a reminder for you to take your medicine.

For an additional supply of these calendars, photocopy the form found in this book.

Filling Out Your Wallet Diary

Fill out your wallet diary with the help of your doctor, nurse, or pharmacist. Then, each time you have an appointment with your doctor, fill in your blood pressure reading so that you can see your progress. Also, enter the date and time for your next visit so that you will not forget. Between visits, write in things to discuss at your next visit so that you can readily recall them at that time.

MEDICATION CALENDAR ②   MONTH AUGUST ← ①

③ Drug Name and Strength

④ Am't

⑤

⑥

Time	Drug Name and Strength	Am't	1 T	2 W	3 TH	4 F	5 SA	6 SU	7 M	8 T	9 W	10 TH	11 F	12 SA	13 SU	14 M	15 T	16 W	17 TH	18 F	19 SA	20 SU	21 M	22 T	23 W	24 TH	25 F	26 SA	27 SU	28 M	29 T	30 W	31 TH
MORNING																																	
8AM	DIURETIC 50 MG	1		✓	✓	✓	✓	✓	✓	✓	✓																						
8AM	PRAZOSIN 2 MG	1		✓	✓	✓	✓	✓	✓	✓	✓																						
AFTERNOON																																	
EVENING																																	
6 PM	DIURETIC 50 MG	1		✓	✓	✓	✓	✓	✓	✓	✓																						
6 PM	PRAZOSIN 2 MG	1		✓	✓	✓	✓	✓	✓	✓	✓																						

EXAMPLE ONLY

MEDICATION CALENDAR

MONTH _____

EVENING						AFTERNOON					MORNING						Time	Drug Name and Strength	Am't	DAY
																				1
																				2
																				3
																				4
																				5
																				6
																				7
																				8
																				9
																				10
																				11
																				12
																				13
																				14
																				15
																				16
																				17
																				18
																				19
																				20
																				21
																				22
																				23
																				24
																				25
																				26
																				27
																				28
																				29
																				30
																				31

MEDICATION CALENDAR

MONTH _____

EVENING AFTERNOON MORNING

Time	Drug Name and Strength	Am't	DAY
			1
			2
			3
			4
			5
			6
			7
			8
			9
			10
			11
			12
			13
			14
			15
			16
			17
			18
			19
			20
			21
			22
			23
			24
			25
			26
			27
			28
			29
			30
			31

MEDICATION CALENDAR

MONTH _____

Time	Drug Name and Strength	Am't	DAY 1	2	3	4	5	6	7	8	9	10	11	12	13	14	15	16	17	18	19	20	21	22	23	24	25	26	27	28	29	30	31

MORNING   AFTERNOON   EVENING

Date	BP	Next Appt.	Things to Discuss at Next Visit

Patient Wallet Diary

—fold—

My Goal BP _____

Name _____

Clinic or MD _____

Telephone _____

Medication:

Instructions:

Patient Wallet Diary

—fold—

My Goal BP _____

Name _____

Clinic or MD _____

Telephone _____

Medication:

Instructions:

Date	BP	Next Appt.	Things to Discuss at Next Visit

Appendix II: NHBPEP Materials for Patients and Consumers

Single copies of patient and consumer pamphlets are available free of charge from the:

National High Blood Pressure Information Center
120/80 National Institutes of Health
Bethesda, Maryland 20892   (301) 473-3260

Name

Organization

Street

City, State, Zip

Phone No. (Include Area Code)

Please check [✔] those publications you are interested in receiving. (Allow four to six weeks for delivery.)

[ ] *High Blood Pressure and What You Can Do About It* Describes nature and measurement of blood pressure, both normal and high, with discussion of drug treatment and side effects as well as recommended lifestyle changes.

[ ] *Questions About Weight, Salt, and High Blood Pressure* Describes what is known about the relationship between certain diet changes and high blood pressure.

[ ] *Blacks and High Blood Pressure* Describes what high blood pressure is, its importance to blacks, the need for treatment, and the role of the patient's family.

[ ] *Verdad Y Ficcion Sobre La Presion Arterial Alta* Designed for a Spanish language audience. Ideal as a handout to anyone getting a blood pressure measurement. Contains basic facts about high blood pressure and corrects some commonly held misconceptions.

Additional publications are currently being developed by NHBPEP. For information about new publications and their availability, check with the National High Blood Pressure Information Center.

Appendix III: Members of the United States Pharmacopeial Convention and the Institutions and Organizations Represented as of July 1, 1988

Current Officers and Board of Trustees

President: Arthur Hull Hayes, Jr., M.D.,* President and Chief Executive Officer, EM Industries, Inc., 5 Skyline Drive, Hawthorne, NY 10532

Vice President: Joseph M. Benforado, M.D.,* 730 Seneca Place, Madison, WI 53711

Past President: Frederick E. Shideman, M.D., Ph.D.,** 4503 Moorland Avenue, Minneapolis, MN 55424

Treasurer: Paul F. Parker, D.Sc.,* Pharmacy Consultant, Paul Parker, Inc., 917 Celia Lane, Lexington, KY 40504

Representing Medicine: J. Richard Crout, M.D.,* Boehringer Mannheim Corporation, 1301 Piccard Drive, Rockville, MD 20850

Leo E. Hollister, M.D., Harris County Psychiatric Center, P.O. Box 20249, Houston, TX 77225

Representing Pharmacy: Joseph P. Buckley, Ph.D.,* College of Pharmacy, 141 SR2, University of Houston, 4800 Calhoun, Houston, TX 77004

James T. Doluisio, Ph.D.,* College of Pharmacy, University of Texas at Austin, Austin, TX 78712

Public Member: Estelle G. Cohen, M.A.* 5813 Greenspring Avenue, Baltimore, MD 21209

At Large: John V. Bergen, Ph.D.,* National Committee for Clinical Laboratory Standards, 771 E. Lancaster Avenue, Villanova, PA 19085

John T. Fay, Jr., Ph.D.,* Bergen Brunswig Corporation, 4000 Metropolitan Drive, Orange, CA 92668

Executive Director and Secretary: William M. Heller, Ph.D.,* 12601 Twinbrook Parkway, Rockville, MD 20852

United States Government Services

Department of the Army: Col. Frank A. Cammarata,* 5111 Leesburg Pike, Falls Church, VA 22041

Department of Health & Human Services: Richard R. Ashbaugh,* 5600 Fishers Lane, Rm. 11-03, Rockville, MD 20857

Food and Drug Administration: Peter H. Rheinstein, M.D., J.D.,* Director, Office of Drug Standards, Center for Drugs and Biologics, 5600 Fishers Lane, HFN-200, Rockville, MD 20857

National Bureau of Standards: Stanley D. Rasberry,* Chemistry, B311, National Bureau of Standards, Gaithersburg, MD 20899

Office of the Chief of Naval Operations, U.S. Navy: Commander Ronnie E. Whiten, MSC, USN, Defense Medical Standardization Board, Fort Detrick, Frederick, MD 21701

Office of the Surgeon General, U.S. Air Force: Lt. Col. John M. Hammond,* USAF/SCB, Bolling AFB, DC 20332

United States Public Health Service: ASG Richard M. Church, 5600 Fishers Lane, Rockville, MD 20857

U.S. Office of Consumer Affairs: Robert F. Steeves, J.D.,* Dep. Spec. Adv. to the President for Consumer Affairs, 1725 I Street, N.W., Suite 1003, Washington, DC 20201

Veterans Administration, Central Office: Stephen M. Sleight, M.Sc.,* Pharmacy Service (119), Veterans Administration Medical Center, Bay Pines, FL 33504

---

*Present at the 1985 Quinquennial Meeting.
**Deceased.

National Organizations

American Association of Pharmaceutical Scientists: Ralph F. Shangraw, Ph.D., University of Maryland, School of Pharmacy, 20 N. Pine Street, Baltimore, MD 21201

American Chemical Society: Samuel M. Tuthill, Ph.D.,* P.O. Box 5439, St. Louis, MO 63147

American Dental Association: Edgar W. Mitchell, Ph.D.,* American Dental Association, 211 E. Chicago Avenue, Chicago, IL 60611

American Hospital Association: William R. Reid, Community Hospital of Roanoke Valley, 101 Elm Avenue, S.E., Box 12946, Roanoke, VA 24029

American Medical Association: John C. Ballin, Ph.D.,* American Medical Association, 535 N. Dearborn Street, Chicago, IL 60610

American Nurses' Association, Inc.: Jean Marshall, B.A., R.N.,* Employee Relations Coordinator, Paul Kimball Hospital, 600 River Avenue, Lakewood, NJ 08701

American Pharmaceutical Association: John F. Schlegel, Pharm.D.,* President, American Pharmaceutical Association, 2215 Constitution Avenue, N.W., Washington, DC 20037

American Society for Clinical Pharmacology & Therapeutics: William B. Abrams, M.D.,* Merck Sharp & Dohme Research Laboratories, West Point, PA 19486

American Society of Hospital Pharmacists: R. David Anderson,* 6 Pelham Greene West, Waynesboro, VA 22980

American Society for Pharmacology & Experimental Therapeutics: Marilyn E. Hess, Ph.D.,* School of Medicine, University of Pennsylvania, Philadelphia, PA 19104

American Society for Quality Control: Theodore C. Fleming,* 7125 Monterrey Drive, Fort Worth, TX 76112

American Veterinary Medical Association: L. Meyer Jones, D.V.M., Ph.D.,* 1225 St. Andrews Drive, Pinehurst, NC 28374

Association of Food and Drug Officials: David R. Work, J.D.,* Executive Director, North Carolina State Board of Pharmacy, P. O. Box H, Carrboro, NC 27510

Association of Official Analytical Chemists: James B. Kottemann,* Food and Drug Administration, 200 C Street, S.W., HFN-004, Washington, DC 20204

Chemical Manufacturers Association: Andrew J. Schmitz, Jr.,* Pfizer, Inc., 235 East 42nd Street, New York, NY 10017

Cosmetic, Toiletry & Fragrance Association, Inc.: G. N. McEwen, Jr., Ph.D., Cosmetic, Toiletry & Fragrance Association, Inc., 1110 Vermont Avenue, N.W., Suite 800, Washington, DC 20005

Health Industry Manufacturers Association: James F. Jorkasky, Director,* Manufacturing & Quality Programs, Health Industry Manufacturers Association, 1030 15th Street, N.W., Washington, DC 20005

National Association of Boards of Pharmacy: Carmen A. Catizone, M.D., R.Ph., Executive Director, National Association of Boards of Pharmacy, O'Hare Corporate Center, 1300 Higgins Road, Suite 103, Park Ridge, IL 60068

National Association of Chain Drug Stores, Inc.: Donald Bell,* Thrift Drug Company, 615 Alpha Drive, Pittsburgh, PA 15230

National Association of Retail Druggists: William N. Tindall, Ph.D.,* 205 Daingerfield Road, Alexandria, VA 22314

National Wholesale Druggists' Association: Ronald J. Streck, Vice President,* Government Affairs, National Wholesale Druggists' Association, 105 Oronoco Street, P. O. Box 238, Alexandria, VA 22313

---

*Present at the 1985 Quinquennial Meeting.

Parenteral Drug Association, Inc.: Sol Motola, Ph.D.,* Bausch & Lomb, Personal Products Division, 1400 North Goodman Street, Rochester, NY 14692

Pharmaceutical Manufacturers Association: John Jennings, M.D.,* Pharmaceutical Manufacturers Association, 1100 Fifteenth Street, N.W., Washington, DC 20005

The Proprietary Association: R. William Soller, Ph.D.,* Vice President, Scientific Affairs, The Proprietary Association, 1150 Connecticut Avenue, N.W. Washington, DC 20036

Other Organizations and Institutions

Alabama

University of Alabama, School of Medicine: Robert B. Diasio, M.D.,* School of Medicine, University of Alabama, Birmingham, AL 35294

University of South Alabama, College of Medicine: Samuel J. Strada, Ph.D., Prof. and Chairman, Dept. of Pharmacology, Univ. of South Alabama, College of Medicine, 3190 MSB, Mobile, AL 36688

Auburn University, School of Pharmacy: Kenneth N. Barker, Ph.D.,* Department of Pharmacy Care Systems, School of Pharmacy, Auburn University, Auburn, AL 36849

Samford University, School of Pharmacy: Stanley V. Susina, Ph.D.,* School of Pharmacy, Samford University, 800 Lakeshore Drive, Birmingham, AL 35229

Medical Association of the State of Alabama: Paul A. Palmisano, M.D.,* Professor of Pediatrics, University of Alabama in Birmingham, University Station, Birmingham, AL 35294

Alaska

Alaska Pharmaceutical Association: Jacqueline L. Warren, 2200 Chinook, Anchorage, AK 99516

Arizona

University of Arizona, College of Med-

icine: Kenneth A. Conrad, M.D., Department of Internal Medicine, College of Medicine, University of Arizona, 1501 North Campbell Avenue, Tucson, AZ 85724

University of Arizona, College of Pharmacy: Samuel H. Yalkowsky, Ph.D.,* College of Pharmacy, University of Arizona, Tucson, AZ 85721

Arizona Pharmacy Association: Mr. Michael J. Henry, 19322 E. Calle de Flors, Queen Creek, AZ 85242

Arkansas

University of Arkansas, College of Medicine: James E. Doherty, III, M.D., VA Hospital, 4300 West 7th Street, Little Rock, AR 72205

University of Arkansas for Medical Sciences, College of Pharmacy: James R. McCowan, Ph.D., College of Pharmacy, University of Arkansas for Medical Sciences, 4301 W. Markham Street, Slot 522, Little Rock, AR 72205

Arkansas Pharmacists Association: Marcus W. Jordin, Ph.D.,* 309 Brookside Drive, Little Rock, AR 72205

California

Loma Linda University, School of Medicine: Ralph E. Cutler, M.D.,* Department of Medicine, Loma Linda School of Medicine, Anderson and Barton, Loma Linda, CA 92354

Stanford University, School of Medicine: Phyllis Gardner, M.D., School of Medicine, Stanford University, CV-291, Stanford, CA 94305

University of California, Davis, School of Medicine: Larry Stark, Ph.D.,* Department of Pharmacology, School of Medicine, University of California, Davis, CA 95616

University of California, Los Angeles, School of Medicine: Don H. Catlin,* Department of Pharmacology, School of Medicine, CHS,

---

*Present at the 1985 Quinquennial Meeting.

University of California, Los Angeles, CA 90024

University of California, San Francisco, School of Medicine: Walter L. Way, M.D.,* Department of Anesthesia, Rm. S-436, University of California, San Francisco, CA 94143

University of Southern California, School of Medicine: Samuel P. Bessman, M.D., MUDD 414, 1333 San Pablo Street, Los Angeles, CA 90033

University of California, San Francisco, School of Pharmacy: Jack Cooper, Ph.D.,* School of Pharmacy, University of California, San Francisco, CA 94143

University of Southern California, School of Pharmacy: Robert T. Koda, Pharm.D., Ph.D.,* School of Pharmacy, University of Southern California, 1985 Zonal Avenue, Los Angeles, CA 90033

University of the Pacific, School of Pharmacy: Alice Jean Matuszak, Ph.D., 751 Brookside Road, Stockton, CA 95207

California Pharmacists Association: Max Stollman,* 8314 Wilshire Boulevard, Beverly Hills, CA 90211

Colorado

University of Colorado, School of Medicine: Antonia Vernadakis, Ph.D., Prof., Depts. of Psych. & Pharm., School of Medicine, University of Colorado, 4200 E. 9th Avenue, Box C263, Denver, CO 80262

University of Colorado, School of Pharmacy: Duane C. Bloedow, Ph.D.,* 3630 Silver Plume Lane, Boulder, CO 80303

Colorado Medical Society: Franklin Lee Bowling, M.D., 1001 E. Oxford Lane, Englewood, CO 80110

Colorado Pharmacal Association: Thomas G. Arthur R. Ph.,* 9852 Corsair Drive, Conifer, CO 80433

Connecticut

University of Connecticut, School of Medicine: Paul F. Davern,* Director of Pharmacy, University of Connecticut Health Center, 261 Farmington Avenue, Farmington, CT 06032

University of Connecticut, School of Pharmacy: Max W. Miller, Ph.D.,* School of Pharmacy, University of Connecticut, Storrs, CT 06268

Connecticut Pharmaceutical Association: Henry A. Palmer, Ph.D.,* 26 Timber Drive, Storrs, CT 06268

Connecticut State Medical Society: James E. O'Brien, M.D., 31 Surrey Drive, Wethersfield, CT 06109

Delaware

Medical Society of Delaware: Jeffry I. Komins, M.D.,* 2323 Pennsylvania Avenue, Wilmington, DE 19806

District of Columbia

Georgetown University, School of Medicine: Arthur Raines, Ph.D., School of Medicine, Georgetown University, 3900 Reservoir Road, N.W., Washington, DC 20007

Howard University, College of Medicine: Robert E. Taylor, M.D., Ph.D., Department of Medicine, Howard University Hospital, 2041 Georgia Avenue, N.W., Washington, DC 20060

Howard University, College of Pharmacy & Pharmacal Sciences: Wendell T. Hill, Jr., Pharm.D.,* 2300 Fourth Street, N.W., Washington, DC 20059

Medical Society of the District of Columbia: Michael D. Abramowitz, M.D.,* 111 Michigan Avenue, N.W., Washington, DC 20010

Florida

Florida A & M University, College of Pharmacy and Pharmaceutical Sciences: Henry Lewis, III, Pharm.D.,* College of Pharmacy and Pharmaceutical Sciences, Florida A & M University, Tallahassee, FL 32307

---

*Present at the 1985 Quinquennial Meeting.

University of Florida, College of Medicine: Thomas F. Muther, Ph.D.,* Department of Pharmacology & Therapeutics, College of Medicine, University of Florida, Box J-267, J. Hillis Miller Health Center, Gainesville, FL 32610

University of Florida, College of Pharmacy: Michael A. Schwartz, Ph.D.,* Box J-4, J. Hillis Miller Health Center, Gainesville, FL 32610

University of South Florida, College of Medicine: Joseph J. Krzanowski, Jr., Ph.D.,* 12901 N. 30th Street, Box 9, Tampa, FL 33612

Florida Pharmacy Association: George Browning,* 8552 Sylvan Drive, Melbourne, FL 32901

Georgia

Medical College of Georgia, School of Medicine: Merle W. Riley, Ph.D.,* Department of Pharmacology & Toxicology, Medical College of Georgia, 1120 Fifteenth Street, Augusta, GA 30912

Mercer University, Southern School of Pharmacy: A. Vincent Lopez, Ph.D.,* Southern School of Pharmacy, Mercer University, 345 Boulevard, N.E., Atlanta, GA 30312

Morehouse School of Medicine: Ralph W. Trottier, Ph.D.,* Morehouse School of Medicine, 720 Westview Drive, S.W., Atlanta, GA 30310

University of Georgia, College of Pharmacy: Howard C. Ansel, Ph.D.,* Dean, College of Pharmacy, University of Georgia, Athens, GA 30602

Georgia Pharmaceutical Association: Charles L. Braucher, Ph.D., College of Pharmacy, University of Georgia, Athens, GA 30602

Medical Association of Georgia: E. D. Bransome, Jr., M.D.,* Professor of Medicine, Medical College of Georgia, Augusta, GA 30912

Idaho

Idaho State University, College of

Pharmacy: Eugene I. Isaacson, Ph.D.,* 1619 East Terry, Pocatello, ID 83201

Illinois

Chicago Medical School/University of Health Sciences: Seymour Ehrenpreis, Ph.D.,* Department of Pharmacology, University of Health Sciences/The Chicago Medical School, 3333 N. Green Bay Road, N. Chicago, IL 60064

Loyola University of Chicago Stritch School of Medicine: John E. Nelson, M.D., Assist. Professor of Medicine, Dept. of Medicine, 2160 S. First Avenue, Maywood, IL 60153

Southern Illinois University, School of Medicine: Ronald A. Browning, Ph.D.,* Department of Medical Physiology and Pharmacology, Southern Illinois University School of Medicine, Carbondale, IL 62901

University of Illinois, College of Medicine: Marten M. Kernis, Ph.D., College of Medicine, University of Illinois, 1853 West Polk Street, Chicago, IL 60612

University of Illinois, College of Pharmacy: Martin I. Blake, Ph.D.,* 9023 Kenton Avenue, Skokie, IL 60076

Illinois Pharmacists Association: Ronald W. Gottrich,* 1817 Clearview Dr., Springfield, IL 62704

Illinois State Medical Society: Vincent A. Costanzo, Jr., M.D.,* 18304 Maple, Lansing, IL 60438

Indiana

Butler University, College of Pharmacy: Margaret A. Shaw, Ph.D.,* College of Pharmacy, Butler University, 4600 Sunset Avenue, Indianapolis, IN 46208

Purdue University, School of Pharmacy and Pharmacal Sciences: Adelbert M. Knevel, Ph.D.,* School of Pharmacy & Pharmacal Sciences, Purdue University, West Lafayette, IN 47907

*Present at the 1985 Quinquennial Meeting.

Indiana State Medical Association: Edward Langston, M.D., 203 North Division, Flora, IN 46924

Iowa

University of Iowa, College of Medicine: John E. Kasik, M.D., Ph.D., Internal Medicine 1A02 VA, University of Iowa, Iowa City, IA 52242

Drake University, College of Pharmacy: Wendell Southard, Ph.D.,* College of Pharmacy, Drake University, Des Moines, IA 50311

University of Iowa, College of Pharmacy: Robert A. Wiley, Ph.D.,* Dean, College of Pharmacy, University of Iowa, Iowa City, IA 52242

Iowa Pharmacists Association: Robert Osterhaus,* 124 S. Main, Maquoketa, IA 52060

Kansas

University of Kansas Medical Center, School of Medicine: Edward J. Walaszek, Ph.D.,* School of Medicine, University of Kansas Medical Center, 39th and Rainbow Boulevard, Kansas City, KS 66103

University of Kansas, School of Pharmacy: Siegfried Lindenbaum, Ph.D.,* 1025 Holiday Drive, Lawrence, KS 66044

Kansas Pharmacists Association: John Owen,* 1202 Eastmoor, Wichita, KS 67207

Kentucky

University of Kentucky, College of Medicine: Edgar T. Iwamoto, Ph.D., College of Medicine, University of Kentucky, Pharmacology, 800 Rose Street, Lexington, KY 40536

University of Kentucky, College of Pharmacy: Patrick P. DeLuca, Ph.D.,* 3292 Nantucket Drive, Lexington, KY 40502

University of Louisville, School of Medicine: Peter P. Rowell, Ph.D.,* Department of Pharmacology & Toxicology, School of Medicine, University of Louisville, Louisville, KY 40292

Kentucky Medical Association: Ellsworth C. Seeley, M.D.,* 820 South Limestone, Annex 4, Lexington, KY 40536

Kentucky Pharmacists Association: Chester L. Parker, Pharm.D.,* 1816 Darien Drive, Lexington, KY 40504

Louisiana

Northeast Louisiana University, School of Pharmacy: Robert D. Kee, Ph.D.,* Turtledove Drive, Monroe, LA 71203

Tulane University, School of Medicine: Floyd R. Domer, Ph.D.,* Department of Pharmacology, School of Medicine, Tulane University, 1430 Tulane Avenue, New Orleans, LA 70112

Xavier University of Louisiana, College of Pharmacy: Josephine Daigle, Ph.D.,* 7325 Palmetto Street, New Orleans, LA 70125

Louisiana Pharmacists Association: William G. Day,* 13114 Country Manor, Baton Rouge, LA 70816

Louisiana State Medical Society: John Adriani, M.D.,* 67 N. Park Place, New Orleans, LA 70124

Maryland

Johns Hopkins University, School of Medicine: E. Robert Feroli, Pharm.D.,* Johns Hopkins Hospital, 600 N. Wolfe Street (526 Osler), Baltimore, MD 21205

Uniformed Services University of the Health Sciences, F. Edward Hebert School of Medicine: Jeffrey D. Lazar, M.D., Department of Pharmacology, USUHS, 4301 Jones Bridge Road, Bethesda, MD 20814

University of Maryland, School of Medicine: James I. Hudson, M.D.,* Dean's Office, School of Medicine, University of Maryland, 655 W. Baltimore Street, Baltimore, MD 21201

*Present at the 1985 Quinquennial Meeting.

University of Maryland, School of Pharmacy: Larry L. Augsburger, Ph.D.,* 20 North Pine Street, Baltimore, MD 21201

Maryland Pharmacists Association: Paul Freiman,* 3 Pipe Hill Court, Baltimore, MD 21209

Massachusetts

Boston University, School of Medicine: Edward W. Pelikan, M.D.,* Department of Pharmacology, Boston University School of Medicine, 80 East Concord Street, Boston, MA 02118

Harvard Medical School: Peter Goldman, M.D., Harvard Medical School, 25 Shattuck Street, Boston, MA 02115

Massachusetts College of Pharmacy & Allied Health Sciences: William O. Foye, Ph.D.,* 179 Longwood Avenue, Boston, MA 02115

Northeastern University, College of Pharmacy and Allied Health Professions: Larry N. Swanson, Pharm.D.,* 124 Cobble Hill Road, Warwick, RI 02886

University of Massachusetts Medical School: Brian Johnson, M.D.,* University of Massachusetts Medical Center, 55 Lake Avenue, North, Worcester, MA 01605

Massachusetts Medical Society: Edward J. Khantzian, M.D., Cambridge Hospital, 1493 Cambridge Street, Cambridge, MA 02139

Massachusetts State Pharmaceutical Association: Bertram A. Nicholas, M.Sc.,* 179 Longwood Avenue, Boston, MA 02115

Michigan

Ferris State College, School of Pharmacy: Gerald W. A. Slywka, Ph.D.,* 7630 Crestview Drive, Reed City, MI 49677

University of Michigan, College of Pharmacy: Ara G. Paul, Ph.D., Dean, College of Pharmacy, University of Michigan, Ann Arbor, MI 48109-1065

Wayne State University, College of Pharmacy and Allied Health Professions: Janardan Nagwekar, Ph.D., College of Pharmacy and Allied Health Professions, Shapero Hall, Room 511, Wayne State University, Detroit, MI 48202

Wayne State University, School of Medicine: Ralph E. Kauffman, M.D.,* 3901 Beaubien, Detroit, MI 48201

Michigan Pharmacists Association: Salvador Pancorbo, Ph.D., Pharm.D.,* College of Pharmacy & Allied Health Professions, Wayne State University, Detroit, MI 48202

Minnesota

University of Minnesota, College of Pharmacy: Edward G. Rippie, Ph.D.,* 2 N. Mallard Road, North Oaks, MN 55127

University of Minnesota Medical School, Minneapolis: Jack W. Miller, Ph.D.,* University of Minnesota Medical School, 3-260 Millard Hall, 435 Delaware Street, S.E., Minneapolis, MN 55455

Minnesota State Pharmaceutical Association: Arnold D. Delger,* 1533 Grantham Street, St. Paul, MN 55108

Mississippi

University of Mississippi, School of Medicine: Richard L. Klein, Ph.D.,* Department of Pharmacology & Toxicology, University of Mississippi Medical Center, Jackson, MS 39216-4504

University of Mississippi, School of Pharmacy: Robert W. Cleary, Ph.D.,* Department of Pharmaceutics, University of Mississippi, University, MS 38677

Mississippi Pharmacists Association: Phylliss M. Moret R.Ph.,* Mississippi Pharmacists Association, 341 Edgewood Terrace Drive, Jackson, MS 39206

---

*Present at the 1985 Quinquennial Meeting.

Missouri

St. Louis College of Pharmacy: John W. Zuzack, Ph.D.,* St. Louis College of Pharmacy, 4588 Parkview Place, St. Louis, MO 63110

St. Louis University, School of Medicine: Alvin H. Gold, Ph.D.,* 1402 S. Grand Boulevard, St. Louis, MO 63104

University of Missouri, Columbia, School of Medicine: John W. Yarbro, M.D., Ph.D.,* N408 Health Sciences Center, Columbia, MO 65212

University of Missouri, Kansas City, School of Medicine: David Rush, Pharm.D.,* Truman Medical Center-East, Little Blue & Lee's Summit Roads, Kansas City, MO 64139

University of Missouri, Kansas City, School of Pharmacy: Wayne M. Brown, Ph.D.,* School of Pharmacy, University of Missouri-Kansas City, 5005 Rockhill Road, Kansas City, MO 64110-2499

Washington University, School of Medicine: H. Mitchell Perry, Jr., M.D.,* School of Medicine, Washington University, Box 8048, 660 S. Euclid Avenue, St. Louis, MO 63110

Missouri Pharmaceutical Association: James R. Boyd, P.D.,* 215 Shirley Ridge Drive, St. Charles, MO 63303

Montana

University of Montana, School of Pharmacy & Allied Health Professions: Donald H. Canham, Ph.D., School of Pharmacy, University of Montana, Missoula, MT 59812

Montana State Pharmaceutical Association: Robert H. Likewise, 4376 Head Drive, Helena, MT 59601

Nebraska

Creighton University, School of Medicine: Michael C. Makoid, Ph.D.,* School of Medicine, Creighton University, 2500 California Street, Omaha, NE 68178

Creighton University, School of Pharmacy and Allied Health Professions: James M. Crampton, Ph.D., School of Pharmacy and Allied Health Professions, Creighton University, California and 24th Streets, Omaha, NE 68178

University of Nebraska, College of Medicine: Manuchair Ebadi, Ph.D., Department of Pharmacology, University of Nebraska, College of Medicine, 42nd Street and Dewey Avenue, Omaha, NE 68105

University of Nebraska, College of Pharmacy: Clarence T. Ueda, Pharm.D., Ph.D., Dean, College of Pharmacy, University of Nebraska, 42nd and Dewey Avenues, Omaha, NE 68105

Nebraska Pharmacists Association: Rex C. Higley, R.P.,* 3110 South 42nd, Lincoln, NE 68506

Nevada

University of Nevada, Reno, School of Medicine: Iain L. O. Buxton, D.Ph.,* Department of Pharmacology, School of Medicine, University of Nevada, Reno, NV 89557

New Hampshire

Dartmouth Medical School: James J. Kresel, Ph.D.,* Dartmouth-Hitchcock Medical Center, Hanover, NH 03756

New Hampshire Pharmaceutical Association: William J. Lancaster,* 4 Woodmore Drive, Hanover, NH 03755

New Jersey

University of Medicine and Dentistry of New Jersey, New Jersey Medical School: Sheldon B. Gertner, Ph.D.,* New Jersey Medical School, UMDNJ, 100 Bergen Street, Newark, NJ 07103

Rutgers, The State University of New Jersey, College of Pharmacy: Thomas Medwick, Ph.D.,* College of Pharmacy, Rutgers, The State

---

*Present at the 1985 Quinquennial Meeting.

University of New Jersey, P. O. Box 789, Piscataway, NJ 08854

Medical Society of New Jersey: Joseph N. Micale, M.D., 914-85th Street, North Bergen, NJ 07047

New Jersey Pharmaceutical Association: Stephen J. Csubak, Ph.D.,* 4 Decision Way East, Washington Crossing, PA 18977

New Mexico

University of New Mexico, College of Pharmacy: William M. Hadley, Ph.D., Dean, College of Pharmacy, University of New Mexico, Albuquerque, NM 87131

New Mexico Pharmaceutical Association: Hugh Kabat, Ph.D.,* College of Pharmacy, University of New Mexico, Albuquerque, NM 87131

New York

Albert Einstein College of Medicine of Yeshiva University: Dr. Walter G. Levine,* Albert Einstein College of Medicine, 1300 Morris Park Avenue, New York, NY 10461

City University of New York, Mt. Sinai School of Medicine: Joel S. Mindel, M.D., Ph.D.,* Department of Ophthalmology, Annenberg Bldg. 22-14, Mt. Sinai School of Medicine, 1 Gustave L. Levy Place, New York, NY 10029

Columbia University College of Physicians and Surgeons: Dr. Norman Kahn,* Department of Pharmacology, Columbia University, 630 West 168th Street, New York, NY 10032

Cornell University Medical College: W. Y. Chan, Ph.D.,* Cornell University Medical College, New York, NY 10021

Long Island University, Arnold and Marie Schwartz College of Pharmacy and Health Sciences: John J. Sciarra, Ph.D.,* 8 Allen Drive, Locust Valley, NY 11560

New York Medical College: Mario A. Inchiosa, Jr., Ph.D.,* Department of Pharmacology, New York Medical College, Valhalla, NY 10595

State University of New York, Buffalo, School of Medicine: Robert J. McIsaac, Ph.D.,* Department of Pharmacology and Therapeutics, School of Medicine, 127 Farber Hall, SUNY at Buffalo, Buffalo, NY 14214

State University of New York, Buffalo, School of Pharmacy: Walter D. Conway, Ph.D., School of Pharmacy, SUNY at Buffalo, H565 Hochstetter Hall, Buffalo, NY 14260

State University of New York, Stony Brook, School of Medicine: Dr. Arthur P. Grollman, Dept. of Pharmacological Science, School of Medicine, SUNY at Stony Brook, BHS T-8 140, Stony Brook, NY 11794

St. John's University, College of Pharmacy and Allied Health Professions: Andrew J. Bartilucci, Ph.D.,* College of Pharmacy and Allied Health Professions, St. John's University, Grand Central and Utopia Parkways, Jamaica, NY 11439

Union University, Albany College of Pharmacy: Barry S. Reiss, Ph.D.,* Albany College of Pharmacy, Union University, 106 New Scotland Avenue, Albany, NY 12208

University of Rochester, School of Medicine and Dentistry: Michael Weintraub, M.D., Ph.D.,* University of Rochester Medical Center, Box 644, Rochester, NY 14642

Medical Society of the State of New York: Richard S. Blum, M.D., 25 Spruce Dr., East Hills, NY 11576

Pharmaceutical Society of the State of New York: Walter Singer, R.Ph., Ph.D., Pharmaceutical Society of the State of New York, Pine West Plaza IV, Washington Avenue Extension, Albany, NY 12205

---

*Present at the 1985 Quinquennial Meeting.

North Carolina

Bowman Gray School of Medicine, Wake Forest University: Jack W. Strandhoy, Ph.D.,* Department of Physiology/Pharmacology, Bowman Gray School of Medicine, Wake Forest University, 300 S. Hawthorne Road, Winston-Salem, NC 27103

Duke University, School of Medicine: William J. Murray, M.D., Ph.D.,* Box 3061, Duke University Medical Center, Durham, NC 27710

East Carolina University, School of Medicine: Wallace R. Wooles, Ph.D. Chairman, Dept. of Pharmacology, School of Medicine, East Carolina University, Greenville, NC 27834

University of North Carolina, Chapel Hill, School of Medicine: Tai-Chan Peng, M.D.,* Department of Pharmacology, School of Medicine, Faculty Laboratory Office Building 231H, University of North Carolina, Chapel Hill, NC 27514

University of North Carolina, Chapel Hill, School of Pharmacy: Richard J. Kowalsky, Pharm.D.,* School of Pharmacy, 24 Beard Hall 200H, University of North Carolina, Chapel Hill, NC 27514

North Carolina Pharmaceutical Association: George H. Cocolas, Ph.D.,* Beard Hall 200H, Chapel Hill, NC 27514

North Dakota

North Dakota State University, College of Pharmacy: William M. Henderson, Ph.D.,* College of Pharmacy, North Dakota State University, Fargo, ND 58105

North Dakota Pharmaceutical Association: William H. Shelver, Ph.D., College of Pharmacy, North Dakota State University, Fargo, ND 58105

Ohio

Case Western Reserve University, School of Medicine: Kenneth A. Scott, Ph.D.,* School of Medicine, Case Western Reserve University, 2119 Abington Road, Cleveland, OH 44106

Medical College of Ohio at Toledo: Robert D. Wilkerson, Ph.D.,* Department of Pharmacology, Medical College of Ohio, 3000 Arlington Avenue, Toledo, OH 43699

Northeastern Ohio University, College of Medicine: Ralph E. Berggren, M.D., Vice Provost for Academic Affairs, College of Medicine, Northeastern Ohio University, Rootstown, OH 44272

Ohio Northern University, College of Pharmacy and Allied Health Sciences: Dr. Ajaz S. Hussain, College of Pharmacy and Allied Health Sciences, Ohio Northern University, Ada, OH 45810

Ohio State University, College of Medicine: Gopi A. Tejwani, Ph.D., Department of Pharmacology, College of Medicine, Ohio State University, 5086 Graves Hall, 333 West 10th Avenue, Columbus, OH 43210-1239

Ohio State University, College of Pharmacy: Michael C. Gerald, Ph.D.,* College of Pharmacy, Ohio State University, 500 West 12th Avenue, Columbus, OH 43210

University of Cincinnati, College of Medicine: Leonard T. Sigell, Ph.D.,* College of Medicine, University of Cincinnati, Rm. 7701, 231 Bethesda Avenue, Mail Location No. 144, Cincinnati, OH 45267-0144

University of Cincinnati, College of Pharmacy: Henry S. I. Tan, Ph.D.,* College of Pharmacy, University of Cincinnati, 136 Health Professions Building, 3223 Eden Avenue, Mail Location No. 4, Cincinnati, OH 45267

University of Toledo, College of Pharmacy: Norman F. Billups, Ph.D., Dean, College of Pharmacy, University of Toledo, Toledo, OH 43606

---

*Present at the 1985 Quinquennial Meeting.

Wright State University, School of Medicine: John O. Lindower, M.D., Ph.D.,* 3301 Stonebridge Road, Kettering, OH 45419

Ohio State Medical Association: Ray W. Gifford, Jr., M.D.,* 3479 Glen Allen Drive, Cleveland, OH 44121

Ohio State Pharmaceutical Association: J. Richard Wuest, Pharm.D.,* 2720 Topichills Drive, Cincinnati, OH 45211

Oklahoma

Oral Roberts University, School of Medicine: Jimmie L. Valentine, Ph.D.,* 8181 South Lewis, Tulsa, OK 74137

Southwestern Oklahoma State University, School of Pharmacy: William G. Waggoner, Ph.D.,* School of Pharmacy, Southwestern Oklahoma State University, 100 Campus Drive, Weatherford, OK 73096

University of Oklahoma, College of Pharmacy: Loyd V. Allen, Jr., Ph.D.,* College of Pharmacy, University of Oklahoma, 1110 N. Stonewall, P. O. Box 26901, Oklahoma City, OK 73190

Oklahoma Pharmaceutical Association: Carl D. Lyons,* Skyline Terrace Nursing Center, 6202 E. 61st, Tulsa, OK 74136

Oklahoma State Medical Association: Clinton Nicholas Corder, M.D., Ph.D.,* 1000 N. Lee, P. O. Box 205, Oklahoma City, OK 73101

Oregon

Oregon Health Sciences University, School of Medicine: Hall Downes, M.D., Ph.D., Pharmacology (SM) L221, Oregon Health Sciences University, Portland, OR 97201

Oregon State University, College of Pharmacy: Freya F. Hermann, College of Pharmacy, Oregon State University, Corvallis, OR 97331

Oregon Medical Association: Richard E. Lahti, M.D.,* 2350 S.W. Multnomah Boulevard, Portland, OR 97219

Oregon State Pharmacists Association: Mrs. Hallie L. Lahti,* 1601 S.E. Oak Shore Lane, Milwaukie, OR 97222

Pennsylvania

Duquesne University, School of Pharmacy: Lawrence H. Block, Ph.D., School of Pharmacy, Mellon Hall of Science, Room 441, Duquesne University, Pittsburgh, PA 15282

Hahnemann University, School of Medicine: Vincent J. Zarro, M.D., Hahnemann University M.S. 431, Broad & Vine Streets, Philadelphia, PA 19102

Medical College of Pennsylvania: Athole G. McNeil Jacobi, M.D., FFARCS,* Medical College of Pennsylvania, 3300 Henry Avenue, Philadelphia, PA 19129

Pennsylvania State University, College of Medicine: John D. Connor, Ph.D.,* Milton S. Hershey Medical Center, Pennsylvania State University, P. O. Box 850, Hershey, PA 17033

Philadelphia College of Pharmacy and Science: Alfonso R. Gennaro, Ph.D.,* Philadelphia College of Pharmacy and Science, 43rd Street and Kingsessing Mall, Philadelphia, PA 19104

Temple University, School of Medicine: Charles A. Papacostas, Ph.D.,* Professor Emeritus, Temple University School of Medicine, 260 North Bent Street, Wyncote, PA 19095

Temple University, School of Pharmacy: Murray Tuckerman, Ph.D.,* School of Pharmacy, Temple University, 3307 N. Broad Street, Philadelphia, PA 19140

Thomas Jefferson University, Jefferson Medical College: C. Paul Bianchi, Ph.D.,* Jefferson Medical College, Thomas Jefferson University, 1020 Locust Street, Philadelphia, PA 19107

---

*Present at the 1985 Quinquennial Meeting.

University of Pennsylvania, School of Medicine: George B. Koelle, M.D., Ph.D., Department of Pharmacology, School of Medicine, University of Pennsylvania, 36th and Hamilton Walk, Philadelphia, PA 19104-6084

University of Pittsburg: Randy P. Juhl, Ph.D., Dean, School of Pharmacy, University of Pittsburg, 1103 Salk Hall, Pittsburgh, PA 15261

University of Pittsburgh, School of Medicine: Robert H. McDonald, Jr., M.D.,* School of Medicine, University of Pittsburgh, 448 Scaife Hall, 3550 Terrace Street, Pittsburgh, PA 15261

Pennsylvania Medical Society: Benjamin Calesnick, M.D.,* 646 W. Springfield Road, Springfield, PA 19064

Pennsylvania Pharmaceutical Association: Joseph A. Mosso R.Ph.,* 319 Carolyn Avenue, Latrobe, PA 15650

Puerto Rico

Ponce School of Medicine: Dr. Arthur L. Hupka, Dept. of Pharmacology, Ponce School of Medicine, P.O. Box 7004, Ponce, PR 00732

Universidad Central del Caribe School of Medicine: Jesús Santos-Martínez, Ph.D., Department of Physiology, School of Medicine, Universidad Central del Caribe, P.O. Box 935, Cayey, PR 00634

University of Puerto Rico, College of Pharmacy: Andrés Malavé, Ph.D., Dean, College of Pharmacy, University of Puerto Rico, G.P.O. Box 5067, San Juan, PR 00936-5067

Rhode Island

Brown University Program in Medicine: Michael C. Wiemann, M.D.,* Roger Williams General Hospital, 825 Chalkstone Avenue, Providence, RI 02908

University of Rhode Island, College of Pharmacy: Christopher Rhodes, Ph.D.,* Department of Pharmaceutics, University of Rhode Island, Kingston, RI 02881

South Carolina

Medical University of South Carolina, College of Medicine: James F. Cooper, Pharm.D., 1056 Fort Sumter Dr., Charleston, SC 29412

Medical University of South Carolina, College of Pharmacy: Paul J. Niebergall, Ph.D.,* Department of Pharmaceutical Sciences, Medical University of South Carolina, 171 Ashley Avenue, Charleston, SC 29425

University of South Carolina, College of Pharmacy: Robert L. Beamer, Ph.D.,* College of Pharmacy, University of South Carolina, Columbia, SC 29208

South Dakota

South Dakota State University, College of Pharmacy: Gary S. Chappell, Ph.D., College of Pharmacy, South Dakota State University, Box 2201, Brookings, SD 57007

Tennessee

East Tennessee State University, Quillen-Dishner College of Medicine: Ernest A. Daigneault, Ph.D.,* 104 Hillside Road, Johnson City, TN 37601

Meharry Medical College, School of Medicine: Dolores C. Shockley, Ph.D.,* Meharry Medical College, 1005 D. B. Todd Boulevard, Nashville, TN 37208

University of Tennessee, College of Medicine: Murray Heimberg, M.D., Ph.D.,* University of Tennessee Center for Health Sciences, 874 Union Avenue, Room 100, Memphis, TN 38163

University of Tennessee, College of Pharmacy: Michael R. Ryan, Ph.D., Dean, College of Pharmacy, University of Tennessee, Center for the Health Sciences, 874 Union Avenue, Room 109, Memphis, TN 38163

---

*Present at the 1985 Quinquennial Meeting.

Texas

Texas Southern University, College of Pharmacy and Health Sciences: Mary Ann Galley, Pharm.D.,* College of Pharmacy and Health Sciences, Texas Southern University, 3100 Cleburne Street, Houston, TX 77004

Texas Tech University, School of Medicine: Thomas W. Hale, Ph.D.,* Texas Tech University Health Science Center, Regional Academic Health Center at Amarillo, 1400 Wallace Boulevard, Amarillo, TX 79106

University of Houston, College of Pharmacy: Joseph P. Buckley, Ph.D.,* College of Pharmacy, University of Houston, 4800 Calhoun Boulevard, Houston, TX 77004

University of Texas, Austin, College of Pharmacy: James T. Doluisio, Ph.D.,* College of Pharmacy, University of Texas at Austin, Austin, TX 78712

University of Texas, Medical School, Galveston: Wayne R. Snodgrass, M.D., Ph.D., Professor of Pediatrics and Pharmacology-Toxicology, University of Texas Medical Branch, Galveston, TX 77550

University of Texas Medical School, Houston: Larry K. Pickering, M.D.,* Medical School at Houston, University of Texas, 6431 Fannin, P. O. Box 20708, Houston, TX 77030

University of Texas Medical School, San Antonio: Arthur H. Briggs, M.D.,* University of Texas Health Science Center at San Antonio, 7703 Floyd Curl Drive, San Antonio, TX 78284

Texas Medical Association: Robert H. Barr, M.D., P.O. Box 25249, Houston, TX 77005

Texas Pharmaceutical Association: Shirley McKee,* P. O. Box 1971, Houston, TX 77251

Utah

University of Utah, College of Pharmacy: Harold H. Wolf, Ph.D., Dean, College of Pharmacy, University of Utah, 201 Skaggs Hall, Salt Lake City, UT 84109

University of Utah, School of Medicine: Douglas E. Rollins, M.D., Ph.D.,* Department of Pharmacology, School of Medicine, University of Utah, 50 N. Medical Drive, Salt Lake City, UT 84132

Utah Pharmaceutical Association: Robert V. Petersen, Ph.D.,* College of Pharmacy, University of Utah, Salt Lake City, UT 84112

Vermont

University of Vermont, College of Medicine: John J. McCormack, Ph.D., Dept. of Pharmacology, College of Medicine, Given Medical Building, University of Vermont, Burlington, VT 05405

Virginia

Eastern Virginia Medical School: Desmond R. H. Gourley, Ph.D.,* Department of Pharmacology, Eastern Virginia Medical School, 700 Olney Road, Norfolk, VA 23501

Medical College of Virginia/Virginia Commonwealth University, School of Medicine: Albert J. Wasserman, M.D., Box 565, MCV Station, Richmond, VA 23298

Medical College of Virginia/Virginia Commonwealth University, School of Pharmacy: William H. Barr, Pharm.D., Ph.D.,* MCV School of Pharmacy, Virginia Commonwealth University, MCV Station Box 581, Richmond, VA 23298-0001

University of Virginia, School of Medicine: Peyton E. Weary, M.D.,* Chairman, Department of Dermatology, School of Medicine, University of Virginia, Box 134-Medical Center, Charlottesville, VA 22908

---

*Present at the 1985 Quinquennial Meeting.

Medical Society of Virginia: William J. Hagood, Jr., M.D.,* P. O. Box 158, Clover, VA 24534

Virginia Pharmaceutical Association: Elmer R. Deffenbaugh, Jr.,* 1407 Cummings Drive, Richmond, VA 23220

Washington

University of Washington, School of Medicine: David W. Johnson, M.D., Director, Area Health Education Ctr., WAMI Regional Programs, School of Medicine, SC-64, University of Washington, Seattle, WA 98195

University of Washington, School of Pharmacy: Lynn R. Brady, Ph.D.,* Asst. Dean, School of Pharmacy, T-341 Health Sciences, SC-69, University of Washington, Seattle, WA 98195

Washington State University, College of Pharmacy: William E. Johnson, Ph.D.,* College of Pharmacy, Washington State University, Pullman, WA 99164-6510

Washington State Pharmacists Association: Danial Baker, College of Pharmacy, WSU-Spokane, W. 601 First Avenue, Spokane, WA 99204

West Virginia

Marshall University, School of Medicine: John L. Szarek, Ph.D., Department of Pharmacology, Marshall University School of Medicine, Huntington, WV 25704-2901

West Virginia University Medical Center, School of Pharmacy: Sidney A. Rosenbluth, Ph.D.,* Dean, School of Pharmacy, West Virginia University Medical Center, Morgantown, WV 26506

West Virginia Pharmacists Association: Art Jacknowitz, Pharm.D.,* 329 Wagner Road, Morgantown, WV 26505

Wisconsin

Medical College of Wisconsin: Richard I. H. Wang, M.D., Ph.D.,* VA Medical Center, 5000 W. National Avenue, Wood, WI 53193

University of Wisconsin, Madison, School of Pharmacy: Chester A. Bond, Pharm.D., School of Pharmacy, University of Wisconsin, Madison, 425 N. Charter Street, Madison, WI 53706

University of Wisconsin Medical School, Madison: Joseph M. Benforado, M.D.,* 730 Seneca Place, Madison, WI 53711

Wisconsin Pharmacists Association: Dennis Dziczkowski,* 11330 W. Woodside Drive, Hales Corners, WI 53130

Wyoming

University of Wyoming, School of Pharmacy: Kenneth F. Nelson, Box 3375, Station, Laramie, WY 82071

Wyoming Pharmaceutical Association: Linda G. Sutherland School of Pharmacy, University of Wyoming, Laramie, WY 82071

Members-at-Large

Norman W. Atwater, Ph.D.,* Box 85, Zion Rd., Hopewell, NJ 08525

Herbert S. Carlin, D.Sc.,* 62 Hilltop Drive, Chappaqua, NY 10514

Lester Chafetz, Ph.D.,* School of Pharmacy, University of Missouri, Kansas City, MO 64110

J. Richard Crout, M.D.,* Boehringer Mannheim Corporation, 1301 Piccard Drive, Rockville, MD 20850

Lloyd E. Davis, D.V.M., Ph.D.,* Professor of Clinical Pharmacology, University of Illinois at Urbana-Champaign, College of Veterinary Medicine, 1102 W. Hazelwood Drive, Urbana, IL 61801

Leroy Fevang, Executive Director, Canadian Pharmaceutical Association, 101 - 1815 Alta Vista, Ottawa, Ontario K1G 3Y6, Canada

Fred T. Mahaffey, Pharm.D., 116 North Hamlin, Park Ridge, IL 60068

---

*Present at the 1985 Quinquennial Meeting.

Stuart L. Nightingale, M.D.,* Associate Commissioner for Health Affairs, Department of Health & Human Services, Public Health Service, Food and Drug Administration, 5600 Fishers Lane, Rockville, MD 20857

Daniel A. Nona, Ph.D.,* Executive Director, The American Council on Pharmaceutical Education, 311 West Superior Street, Chicago, IL 60610

Mark Novitch, M.D.,* The Upjohn Company, Kalamazoo, MI 49001

Donald O. Schiffman, Ph.D.,* Secretary, United States Adopted Names Council, 535 North Dearborn Street, Chicago, IL 60610

Albert L. Sheffer, M.D.,* 110 Francis Street, Boston, MA 02215

Eugene A. Timm, Ph.D.,* Immuno-U.S., Inc., 1200 Parkdale Road, Rochester, MI 48063

Carl E. Trinca, Ph.D.,* Executive Director, American Association of Colleges of Pharmacy, 1426 Prince Street, Alexandria, VA 22314

Lawrence C. Weaver, Ph.D.,* Vice President, Professional Relations, Pharmaceutical Manufacturers Association, 1100 Fifteenth Street, N.W., Washington, DC 20005

Members-at-Large (Representing Other Countries That Provide Legal Status To USP or NF)

Salman A. Alfarsi, Ph.D., General Director, General Laboratories and Blood Bank, Saudi Arabia

Thomas D. Arias, Ph.D.,* Departamento del Investigación y Docencia, Universidad de Panamá, Apartado Postal 10767, Estafeta Universitaria, Panamá, Republica de Panamá

Denys Cook, Ph.D.,* Director, Drug Research Laboratories, Health Protection Branch, Tunney's Pasture, Ottawa, Ontario, K1A 0L2, Canada

Quintin L. Kintanar, M.D., Ph.D., Deputy Director General, National Science & Technology Authority, Bicutan, Taguig, Philippines

Kun Ho Yong, Director, Department of Safety Research, NIH, Republic of Korea, 5 Nokbun-Dong, Eunpyung-Ku, Seoul, 122, Korea

Members-at-Large (Public)

Estelle G. Cohen, M.A.* 5813 Greenspring Avenue, Baltimore, MD 21209

Alexander Grant,* Associate Commissioner for Consumer Affairs, Department of Health & Human Services, Public Health Service, Food and Drug Administration, Parklawn Bldg., Room 16-85, 5600 Fishers Lane, Rockville, MD 20857

Paul G. Rogers,* Chairman of the Board, National Council on Patient Information & Education, 1526 I Street, N.W., Washington, DC 20006

Frances M. West,* Secretary, State of Delaware, Department of Community Affairs, 156 South State Street, P. O. Box 1401, Dover, DE 19901

Ex-Officio Members

William H. Barr, Pharm.D., Ph.D., School of Pharmacy, Medical College of Virginia, Health Sciences Div. of VCU, Richmond, VA 23219

Peter Goldman, M.D., Food and Drug Laboratory, 665 Huntington Avenue, Boston, MA 02115

Felix B. Gorrell, 5035 35th Road N., Arlington, VA 22207

William J. Kinnard, Jr., Ph.D.,* Dean, School of Pharmacy, University of Maryland, 20 North Pine Street, Baltimore, MD 21201

Irwin Lerner, President and Chief Executive Officer, Hoffmann-La-Roche, Inc., Nutley, NJ 07110

John A. Owen, Jr., M.D.,* Box 242, University of Virginia Hospital, Charlottesville, VA 22901

Harry C. Shirkey, M.D.,* 1216 Paxton Avenue, Cincinnati, OH 45208

---

*Present at the 1985 Quinquennial Meeting.

Committee Chairmen

Credentials Committee: Peyton E. Weary, M.D., Chairman, Dept. of Dermatology, School of Medicine, University of Virginia, Box 134 Medical Center, Charlottsville, VA 22908

Nominating Committee for the General Committee of Revision: Klaus G. Florey, Ph.D.,* Squibb Institute for Medical Research, P. O. Box 191, New Brunswick, NJ 08903

Nominating Committee for Officers and Trustees: Ray W. Gifford, M.D.,* 3479 Glen Allen Drive, Cleveland Heights, OH 44121

Resolutions Committee: Arthur Hull Hayes, Jr., M.D.,* President and Chief Executive Officer, EM Industries, Inc., 5 Skyline Drive, Hawthorne, NY 10532

General Committee of Revision: William M. Heller, Ph.D.,* 12601 Twinbrook Parkway, Rockville, MD 20852

Honorary Members

George F. Archambault, Pharm.D., J.D.,* 5916 Melvern Drive, Bethesda, MD 20817

Lloyd C. Miller, Ph.D.,* 1625 Skyhawk Road, Escondido, CA 92025

Harry C. Shirkey, M.D.,* 1216 Paxton Avenue, Cincinnati, OH 45208

---

*Present at the 1985 Quinquennial Meeting.

Index

Index

Brand names are in *italics*. There are many brands and different manufacturers of drugs and the listing of selected American and Canadian brand names and manufacturers is intended only for ease of reference. There are additional brands and manufacturers that have not been included. The inclusion of a brand name does not mean the USPC has any particular knowledge that the brand listed has properties different from other brands of the same drug, nor should it be interpreted as an endorsement by the USPC. Similarly, the fact that a particular brand has not been included does not indicate that the product has been judged to be unsatisfactory or unacceptable.

A

B–C

D–G

M–O

P–S

T–Z